Resuscitation

Editor

ANDREW M. MCCOY

CARDIOLOGY CLINICS

www.cardiology.theclinics.com

August 2018 • Volume 36 • Number 3

ELSEVIER

1600 John F. Kennedy Boulevard • Suite 1800 • Philadelphia, Pennsylvania, 19103-2899

http://www.theclinics.com

CARDIOLOGY CLINICS Volume 36, Number 3
August 2018 ISSN 0733-8651, ISBN-13: 978-0-323-61382-8

Editor: Stacy Eastman
Developmental Editor: Sara Watkins

Cardiology Clinics (ISSN 0733-8651) is published quarterly by Elsevier Inc., 360 Park Avenue South, New York, NY 10010-1710. Months of issue are February, May, August, and November. Business and Editorial Offices: 1600 John F. Kennedy Blvd., Ste. 1800, Philadelphia, PA 19103-2899. Customer Service Office: 3251 Riverport Lane, Maryland Heights, MO 63043. Periodicals post-age paid at New York, NY and additional mailing offices. Subscription prices are $339.00 per year for US individuals, $640.00 per year for US institutions, $100.00 per year for US students and residents, $430.00 per year for Canadian individuals, $804.00 per year for Canadian institutions, $464.00 per year for international individuals, $804.00 per year for international institutions and $220.00 per year for Canadian and international students/residents. To receive student/resident rate, orders must be accompanied by name of affiliated institution, data of term, and the *signature* of program/residency coordinator on institution letterhead. Orders will be billed at individual rate until proof of status is received. Foreign air speed delivery is included in all *Clinics* subscription prices. All prices are subject to change without notice. **POSTMASTER:** Send address changes to *Cardiology Clinics*, Elsevier Health Sciences Division, Subscription Customer Service, 3251 Riverport Lane, Maryland Heights, MO 63043. **Customer Service: 1-800-654-2452 (U.S. and Canada); 314-447-8871 (outside U.S. and Canada). Fax: 314-447-8029. E-mail: journalscustomerservice-usa@ elsevier.com (for print support); journalsonlinesupport-usa@elsevier.com (for online support).**

Reprints. For copies of 100 or more, of articles in this publication, please contact the Commercial Reprints Department, Elsevier Inc., 360 Park Avenue South, New York, NY 10010-1710. Tel.: 212-633-3874; Fax: 212-633-3820; E-mail: reprints@elsevier.com.

Cardiology Clinics is also published in Spanish by McGraw-Hill Interamericana Editores S. A., P.O. Box 5-237, 06500, Mexico D. F., Mexico; in Portuguese by Reichmann and Alfonso Editores Rio de Janeiro, Brazil; and in Greek by Dimitrios P. Lagos, 8 Pondon Street, GR115-28 Ilissia, Greece.

Cardiology Clinics is covered in *MEDLINE/PubMed (Index Medicus)*, *Excerpta Medica*, *The Cumulative Index to Nursing and Allied Health Literature* (CINAHL).

Contributors

RAVI S. HIRA, MD
Department of Medicine, Division of
Cardiology, University of Washington,
Harborview Medical Center, Seattle,
Washington, USA

NICHOLAS J. JOHNSON, MD
Assistant Professor, Department of Emergency
Medicine, Adjunct Assistant Professor,
Division of Pulmonary, Critical Care, and Sleep
Medicine, University of Washington,
Harborview Medical Center, Seattle,
Washington, USA

SAMAN KASHANI, MD, MSc
Los Angeles Fire Department, EMS Bureau,
Division of Emergency Medical Services, EMS
Fellow, Department of Emergency Medicine,
Keck School of Medicine of USC, Los Angeles,
California, USA

KATHLEEN KEARNEY, MD
Department of Medicine, Division of
Cardiology, University of Washington, Seattle,
Washington, USA

DAVID H. LAM, MD
Department of Medicine, Division of
Cardiology, University of Washington, Seattle,
Washington, USA

ANDREW J. LATIMER, MD
Senior Fellow, Acting Instructor, Department of
Emergency Medicine, University of
Washington, Seattle, Washington, USA

CHRISTIAN MARTIN-GILL, MD, MPH
Assistant Professor, Department of
Emergency Medicine, University of Pittsburgh
School of Medicine, Pittsburgh, Pennsylvania,
USA

ANDREW M. McCOY, MD, MS
Acting Assistant Professor, Department
of Emergency Medicine, University of
Washington, Resuscitation Academy,
Medical Director, American Medical Response,
Puget Sound Operations, Medical Director,
Shoreline Fire Department, Seattle,
Washington, USA

CLAIRE A. NORDEEN, MD
Emergency Medical Services Fellow,
Department of Emergency Medicine,
University of Washington, Harborview Medical
Center, Seattle, Washington, USA

ESSIE REED-SCHRADER, MD
EMS Fellow, Department of Emergency
Medicine, University at Buffalo, Buffalo,
New York, USA

WILLIAM T. RIVERS, MD
EMS Fellow, Department of Emergency
Medicine, University at Buffalo, Buffalo, New
York, USA

STEPHEN SANKO, MD
Los Angeles Fire Department, EMS Bureau,
Division of Emergency Medical Services,
Assistant Professor, Department of Emergency
Medicine, Keck School of Medicine of USC,
Los Angeles, California, USA

TIMOTHY SATTY, MD
Emergency Medicine Resident, Department of
Emergency Medicine, University of Pittsburgh
School of Medicine, Pittsburgh, Pennsylvania,
USA

MICHAEL R. SAYRE, MD
Professor, Department of Emergency
Medicine, University of Washington, Medical
Director, Seattle Fire Department, Seattle,
Washington, USA

ERICA M. SIMON, DO, MHA
Military Emergency Medical Services and
Disaster Medicine Fellow, Department of
Emergency Medicine, San Antonio Uniformed
Services Health Education Consortium, Fort
Sam Houston, Texas, USA

KAREN SMITH, PhD
Director, Centre for Research and Evaluation,
Ambulance Victoria, Departments of
Epidemiology and Preventive Medicine, and
Community Emergency Health and Paramedic
Practice, Monash University, Melbourne,
Victoria, Australia

HOLBROOK HILL STOECKLEIN, MD
Salt Lake City Fire Department, Division of
Emergency Medicine, Adjunct Faculty,
Department of Surgery, University of Utah,
University of Utah School of Medicine, Salt
Lake City, Utah, USA

DION STUB, MBBS, PhD
Interventional Cardiologist, Department
of Epidemiology and Preventive
Medicine, Monash University,
Cardiology Department, Alfred Hospital,
Western Health, Medical Directorate,
Ambulance Victoria, Melbourne, Victoria,
Australia

KAORI TANAKA, DO, MSPH
Assistant Professor, Department of
Emergency Medicine, Emergency
Medical Services Fellowship Associate
Program Director, Director of Special
Operations, UT Health San Antonio,
San Antonio, Texas, USA

AMY C. WALKER, MD
Resident, Department of Emergency Medicine,
University of Washington, Harborview Medical
Center, Seattle, Washington, USA

LYNN J. WHITE, MS
National Director of Clinical Practice, American
Medical Response, Greenwood Village,
Colorado, USA

**SCOTT T. YOUNGQUIST, MD, MS, FACEP,
FAEMS, FAHA**
Medical Director, Salt Lake City Fire
Department, Division of Emergency Medicine,
Associate Professor, Department of Surgery,
University of Utah, University of Utah School of
Medicine, Salt Lake City, Utah, USA

Contents

Creating a system of care for out-of-hospital cardiac arrest (OHCA) is not a simple task. It must be a multifaceted approach that encompasses a variety of teams from call takers, to bystanders, to emergency medical service (EMS) personnel, to hospital personnel. All of these teams must line up and perform their individual task successfully to yield a survivor of OHCA and return a loved one to his or her family. Various best practices have been collected and are highlighted here. Implementation of these concepts in one's system of care for OHCA is not easy but will result in a greater number of survivors returning to their family in the community.

 Audio content accompanies this article at http://www.cardiology.theclinics.com.

There are 240 million 9-1-1 calls in the United States every year. The burden of managing these emergencies until first responders can arrive is on the dispatchers working in the 5806 public safety answering points, more commonly known as dispatch centers. They are the first link in the chain of survival between the public and the remainder of the health care system. Dispatchers play a critical role in the early identification of emergencies, assignment of appropriate emergency resources, and provision of life-sustaining interventions such as dispatcher-assisted cardiopulmonary resuscitation and disaster management.

Much of the current evidence and many of the recent treatment recommendations for increasing survival from cardiac arrest revolve around improving the quality of cardiopulmonary resuscitation during resuscitation. A focus on providing treatments proved beneficial, and providing these treatments reliably, using measurement, monitoring, and implementation of quality-improvement strategies, will help eliminate variation in outcomes and provide a foundation from which future improvements in resuscitation care can be developed. Using the knowledge and tools available at present will help reduce the ambiguity and variability that exists in resuscitation and provide the ability to save more lives in communities.

Managing out-of-hospital cardiac arrest involves unique challenges, including delays in the initiation of advanced interventions and a limited number of trained personnel on scene. Recent out-of-hospital randomized controlled trials, systematic reviews, and meta-analyses provide key insights into what interventions are best proven to positively affect patient outcomes from out-of-hospital cardiac arrest. The authors review the literature on medications used in out-of-hospital cardiac arrest and summarize evidence-based guidelines from the American Heart Association that form the basis for most emergency medical services cardiac arrest protocols across the United States.

High-quality cardiopulmonary resuscitation, in particular chest compressions, is a key aspect of out-of-hospital cardiac arrest (OHCA) resuscitation. Manual chest compressions remain the standard of care; however, the extrication and transport of patients with OHCA undermine the quality of manual chest compressions and risk the safety of paramedics. Therefore, in circumstances in which high-quality manual chest compressions are difficult or unsafe, paramedics should consider using a mechanical device. By combining high-quality manual chest compressions and judicious application of mechanical chest compressions, emergency medical service agencies can optimize paramedic safety and patient outcomes.

Cardiopulmonary resuscitation (CPR) quality, including chest compression rate, depth, and fraction of hands-on time, is integral to cardiac arrest survival. Introducing mechanized devices to target these measures of quality in the challenging prehospital environment holds great promise. On comparison of mechanical with manual CPR, animal models deliver favorable results on markers of perfusion and manikin studies demonstrate improved consistency of high-quality CPR performance with device use. Factoring in real-world application with prospective randomized human trials, however, repeatedly fails to show improvements in patient-centered outcomes and thus cannot be supported by current scientific evidence.

Ventricular fibrillation (VF) is the most commonly encountered arrhythmia following out-of-hospital cardiac arrest. Previous studies have demonstrated early defibrillation and bystander cardiopulmonary resuscitation as essential in reducing patient mortality. What remains a clinical concern, however, is the treatment of patients experiencing VF refractory to defibrillation. Although current guidelines advocate pharmacotherapy for the management of shock-refractory VF, double sequential defibrillation has become a popular topic of discussion. This article provides a discourse regarding refractory VF and a review of the double sequential defibrillation literature. Further study is required before the recommendation for widespread implementation of this defibrillation technique.

 Video content accompanies this article at www.cardiology.theclinics.com.

Ventricular fibrillation is a life-threatening cardiac arrhythmia that leads to a loss of cardiac function and sudden cardiac death. In this article, the authors summarize therapeutic interventions and guidelines for providers managing patients with out-of-hospital cardiac arrest and refractory ventricular fibrillation in prehospital and emergency settings. In addition, the authors review invasive management, including urgent coronary angiography, extracorporeal membrane oxygenation, and novel strategies for managing refractory ventricular fibrillation arrest. Although the majority of patients with refractory VF do not respond to conventional therapy, recent trials of novel strategies demonstrate encouraging results.

Survival for out-of-hospital cardiac arrest (OHCA) is, on average, approximately 10%, but considerable variability exists among emergency medical services (EMS) systems across the United States. The medical director of an EMS system has considerable control and influence over outcomes in a system by developing evidence-based protocols and overseeing a robust system of quality assurance. A vision for system-level oversight of care that includes continuous data collection and assessment, personally delivered and constructive feedback to providers, and a constant drive for improvement can result in improvements in both processes and patient-centered outcomes.

The post–cardiac arrest syndrome is a highly inflammatory state characterized by organ dysfunction, systemic ischemia and reperfusion injury, and persistent precipitating pathology. Early critical care should focus on identifying and treating the causes of arrest and minimizing further injury to the brain and other organs by optimizing perfusion, oxygenation, ventilation, and temperature. Patients should be treated with targeted temperature management, although the exact temperature goal is not clear. No earlier than 72 hours after rewarming, prognostication using a multimodal approach should inform discussions with families regarding likely neurologic outcome.

The care for survivors of out-of-hospital cardiac arrest is evolving and will be influenced by future and emerging technologies that will play a role in the systems of care for these patients. Recent advances in extracorporeal life support and point-of-care ultrasound imaging, both in-hospital and out-of-hospital, may offer a therapeutic solution in some systems for patients with refractory or recurrent cardiac arrest. Drones capable of delivering automated external defibrillators to the scene of an out-of-hospital cardiac arrest, advances in digital and mobile technologies to notify and leverage bystander response, and wearable life detection technologies may improve survival.

CARDIOLOGY CLINICS

THE CLINICS ARE AVAILABLE ONLINE!
Access your subscription at:
www.theclinics.com

Preface
A Window into Cutting Edge Prehospital Care of the Cardiac Arrest Patient

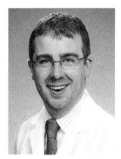

Andrew M. McCoy, MD, MS
Editor

The vast majority of patients who will be treated for cardiac arrest will have their initial arrest prior to arriving at the hospital. Most of these patients will receive treatment from Emergency Medical Services (EMS), and yet most practicing physicians have little to no knowledge of how this care is organized and provided. The genesis of this issue of *Cardiology Clinics* is to address exactly that gap and allow the reader to acquire a detailed knowledge of best practices as well as some controversy in the treatment of out-of-hospital cardiac arrest.

I hope that reviewing this issue will lead you to honestly consider what you know about the EMS system where you care for patients. Many of the concepts may be new to the reader, and each article contained herein is an excellent introduction to a topic that will affect the patients you care for in the hospital as well as a set that did not make it that far. Please probe further. Ask the difficult questions in your system; seek improvement wherever you can. Get involved, whether it is educating your local EMS providers, providing them feedback, or simply patting them on the back and thanking them for their hard work after a difficult case. These moments will lead to improved patient outcomes; they will lead to more cardiac arrest patients returning home to their family.

This primer will get you hooked on prehospital care, but the people who provide that care will keep you coming back for more. Their thirst for knowledge and direction in the care of the sickest of patients is never-ending. To the extent that you can quench that thirst, please have at it. You will find nothing but the best of humanity in these providers, and they will relish the opportunity to learn from you. Systems with close integration between multiple specialties, including Cardiology, Critical Care, Emergency Medicine, and Prehospital care teams, are those that have superior outcomes from out-of-hospital cardiac arrest.

I would like to extend my deepest gratitude to the editors and staff at *Cardiology Clinics*, without whom this issue would not have been possible. Their talent and dedication allowed this issue to flourish.

Andrew M. McCoy, MD, MS
Department of Emergency Medicine
University of Washington
American Medical Response
Puget Sound Operations
Shoreline Fire Department
Harborview Medical Center
325 9th Avenue
Box 359702
Seattle, WA 98104, USA

E-mail address:
mccoya2@uw.edu

Cardiol Clin 36 (2018) xi
https://doi.org/10.1016/j.ccl.2018.04.001
0733-8651/18/© 2018 Published by Elsevier Inc.

Ten Steps to Improve Cardiac Arrest Survival in Your Community

Andrew M. McCoy, MD, MS[a,b,*]

KEYWORDS

- Cardiac arrest • System improvement • Out of hospital cardiac arrest • Registry
- Telecommunicator cardiopulmonary resuscitation • Culture of excellence

KEY POINTS

- Improving successful resuscitation from out of hospital cardiac arrest (OHCA) begins at the call for help.
- Once on scene, professional rescuers should perform high-performance cardiopulmonary resuscitation (CPR), with measurement and postevent feedback, as well as registry collection of their efforts and results to better system-wide performance improvement efforts.
- First responders, including police, should be leveraged to create a system where early chest compressions and defibrillation are paramount.
- Advanced technologies may assist with various elements of OHCA care, and teaching CPR in schools will increase the likelihood that lay persons are comfortable performing CPR when needed.
- Accountability is a key portion of the creation of a culture of excellence within a system of care for OHCA.

INTRODUCTION

The goal of every system of care for patients with out of hospital cardiac arrest (OHCA) is to generate survivors. Some systems succeed more often than others. From these successful systems, lessons can be developed around best practices and recommendations for strategies that have succeeded in the past. These lessons have been collected over the years and developed into a curriculum that is taught as the Resuscitation Academy. This article is a brief overview of some of what one would encounter when attending a Resuscitation Academy.

The tendency for the reader will be to think, "ya, we do that." Please, read in detail the recommendations/best practices and verify that you actually "do that." Go to your dispatch center and see how they dispatch a cardiac arrest. Take a stopwatch and time it, either surreptitiously or overtly. Find out which registry you use and how you use it. Most emergency medical services (EMS) systems do not fully complete many of these steps, although they may touch on the ideas here.

Throughout this reading, you will notice several phrases in italicized bold writing. These are the mantras. These sayings come up over and over again in the Resuscitation Academy. Some are self-evident, but most consist of multiple levels of complexity. These brief words should help to inspire in times of difficulty in implementing a system to care for OHCA patients. These words are proof that others have come before, have seen similar difficulties, and have been able to drive

Disclosures: The author claims no disclosures.
a Department of Emergency Medicine, University of Washington, 325 9th Avenue, Seattle, WA 98104, USA;
b Resuscitation Academy, Seattle, WA, USA
* Harborview Medical Center, Box 359702, 325 9th Avenue, Seattle, WA 98104-2499.
E-mail address: mccoya2@uw.edu

Cardiol Clin 36 (2018) 335–342
https://doi.org/10.1016/j.ccl.2018.03.011

past, significantly improving survival in their community. You can do it, too.

CARDIAC ARREST REGISTRY

The primary mantra of the Resuscitation Academy, the phrase one would hear over and over again when in attendance, is *Measure and Improve*. The concept is that when measuring aspects of care in a system, the improvements that are needed flow naturally and become evident. Stated differently, success cannot be determined until it is defined and tracked. With a definition of success, progress can be measured from current state to a desired state, and the process can be improved to produce the desired outcome.

A prime area where this occurs is in cardiac arrest systems of care. It is truly difficult to improve a system until one is measuring the status quo. Registries have existed for years, first on paper, then in rudimentary form on computers, in spreadsheets, and now in more complex and flexible databases. The largest OHCA registry in the United States is the Cardiac Arrest Registry to Enhance Survival, or CARES (mycares.net). CARES allows for entry, recording, measurement, analysis, and comparison of many aspects of the care provided to patients with OHCA including telecommunicator variables, prehospital variables, patient variables, in-hospital data, and patient outcome information, where available. These data are aggregated in a privacy-centric way and may be benchmarked against other similar systems and national averages. Furthermore, CARES has worked to spread internationally and make data collection tools useful in other countries.

The benefits of a registry to collect data and allow for its analysis in a system of care for OHCA are multiple. A registry allows for large-scale feedback to teams on the overall direction of the program (eg, cardiopulmonary resuscitation [CPR] fraction has increased from an average of 70% to 92%). Discussing registry data with EMS crews also appears to have a version of a Hawthorne effect; once crews know their work is being watched, they seem to try even harder for their patients and are increasingly receptive to feedback as they receive nonpunitive feedback on their performance. Additionally, data from a registry can be analyzed to give receiving hospitals information about their performance and to ensure the hospital and other stakeholders that the EMS system is performing at a high level or working to improve.

Lessons learned from those systems that have implemented registries are important to consider. These include the notion that entering registry data is best completed when it is an assigned duty for a person. This provides accountability and ensures completion of the data. While enrolling in a registry and assigning a person to be responsible for data entry is resource intensive, it is highly likely to pay dividends down the road for an organization that is seeking improvement in its system of care for OHCA.

TELECOMMUNICATOR CARDIOPULMONARY RESUSCITATION

When a lay person calls a central authority for emergency assistance, in many communities there is an attempt to provide instructions to the caller to assist the person in distress while professional aid is in route. This aid is proven to save lives in the treatment of OHCA.[1] In some of these call centers, these activities are measured and put through a quality improvement process. Feedback may even be provided to call takers to assist in their improvement in delivering prearrival aid.

Broadly, many problems exist in systems of care for patient prior to arrival of emergency aid. In order to provide CPR instructions, the telecommunicator must recognize cardiac arrest in a time-efficient manner and provide concise, clear instructions to the caller with regard to patient positioning and the delivery of chest compressions. Several of these steps can break down. For example, callers who speak a different language than the call taker can cause significant delays. The diagnosis can be missed or overdiagnosis can be sought. Overdiagnosis in this case is seeking an etiology by the call taker when only the need for CPR is indicated. If the patient needs CPR, the etiology can wait. Some caller interrogation systems in place delay compressions while seeking an etiology. The approach recommended by faculty in the Resuscitation Academy is that of *No… No… Go…*. In this approach to caller interrogation, once an address is established, the caller is asked if the patient is awake and if the patient is breathing normally. If the answer to both of these questions is no, CPR instructions are immediately initiated. Occasionally, CPR is provided unnecessarily; however, it is then stopped quickly, and little harm has been shown to occur to these patients.[2]

The American Heart Association has recently put out program recommendations and performance measures to help optimize telecommunicator CPR.[3] Adopting many, or potentially all, of these best practices can lead to a high performing telecommunicator CPR system that will predictably yield an increase in survivors in an EMS system.

High-quality feedback to these call takers is integral to ensuring the success of a telecommunicator CPR program. This feedback can include metrics such as percent recognition of cardiac arrest, percent of calls with CPR instructions delivered, time to recognition of cardiac arrest, and time to first chest compression. Cardiac arrest represents a small fraction of all calls to emergency telecommunicators. As the leader of a program, access these calls, listen to them, provide feedback on them. The dividends will be multiple, and your system of care will improve. The cost of a poorly performing telecommunicator CPR system is time; it will take longer for CPR to start, and fewer patients will survive their cardiac arrest.

HIGH-PERFORMANCE CARDIOPULMONARY RESUSCITATION

Created on the back of a napkin in Seattle by a group of firefighter paramedics who wanted to codify the improvements made to CPR training and execution, high-performance CPR (HPCPR), as it would later be named, is more than chest compressions. HPCPR stops the dying process. Effective CPR allows time for other interventions to assist in revering the process of dying. This approach to the scene of care at the side of a cardiac arrest patient is based on tenets that enable optimal care.

The first of these tenets is that the basic life support (BLS) providers, the emergency medical technicians (EMTs), whose team is providing the CPR, own the resuscitation. Too often in OHCA care, the advanced providers swoop in and throw off the resuscitation. CPR pauses lengthen as attempts at difficult advanced skills take longer than expected. In HPCPR, the BLS providers are empowered to take charge and ensure that the patient receives the basic interventions that required while advanced interventions are performed around the basic skills with a minimum of interruptions. BLS owns CPR.

The second tenet is that performance standards should be established, and training should aim for those standards. The faculty of the Resuscitation Academy are strong believers in *Performance not Protocol*. This is the concept that the execution of the team plan, a shared mental model, is more important than the content of that plan. For example, it has not been proven to change outcome if epinephrine is dosed in 0.5 mg or 1 mg increments,[4] but the confusion around a provider unexpectedly calling for an uncommon dose is likely to throw off the entire resuscitation such that deleterious delays may occur, and confusion may intercede and prevent successful resuscitation. Have a well thought out plan and stick to it. This should include standards around training, such as a goal rate for chest compressions. Telling

a provider 100 to 120 compressions per minute is not providing a goal; instead tell a specific number, say 110. Train to 110; provide a metronome that has an audible signal for 110, and finally provide feedback to let the provider know if he or she actually performed at 110 beats per minute. When given a goal, human nature will prevail, and those who seek to provide optimal care will meet the expectations set out for them.

The final tenet is to celebrate successes. When HPCPR works, the number of survivors in a community will increase. Tell these stories to the providers. Let them know that their hard efforts resulted in a community member returning to work, returning to their family. Link these survivors, if willing, with the care providers who resuscitated them. Through celebrating successes, the desire to create survivors will become infectious among the providers.

For more details on the best science surrounding CPR, including a thorough understanding of the biochemical nature of the processes at hand and the overall process variables of importance, a recent review paper is suggested.[5] This paper will also assist the reader in a thorough understanding of the standards around HPCPR and their scientific basis.

RAPID DISPATCH

It would seem logical that the wheels on a first response vehicle would roll as soon as a verified address and a known need for help are established by a call taker at an emergency call center. This idea, simplified with the term rapid dispatch, is not ubiquitous and is not easy to perform for the call taker or the standard programs with which they perform their job. Prioritization of this concept, however, can lead to real and significant improvements in survival from out of hospital cardiac arrest.

It takes a system to save a victim. The first steps in that system revolve around the call for emergency assistance. Call takers, if given the freedom to do so, can often identify very early in the call that assistance is needed. In a system built on BLS first response, followed by a layer of ALS if required, wheels on a BLS vehicle moving toward the scene of an emergency as soon as possible is optimal. Of note, this concept does not require the recognition of cardiac arrest or some other etiology of the call to initiate a response. Instead, the concept relies on the trained emergency telecommunicator to initiate a response as soon as he or she knows help is needed. Empowering these professionals to act when they know help is needed rather than requiring a precise etiology before action can be initiated is preferred.

Attempts have been made to quantify the difference from early allocation of emergency assets. Nichol and colleagues[6] examined the activation interval, or time from call pick up to notification of EMS providers to respond to a call. In their analysis, cutting 30 seconds off of the activation time resulted in a 0.7% survival rate increase independent of other factors associated with the arrest. Furthermore, patients with briefer intervals (<1 min vs >1.5 min) were 69% more likely to survive to hospital discharge. Finally, shorter activation intervals were more impactful on survival than shorter response times (notification of call to arrival on scene).

Understanding the inner workings of the local 911 call centers is integral to the success of a system of care for OHCA. Making significant change early in the chain of care for OHCA can lead to large gains on the back end; ensuring that this happens in your local 911 call center whenever appropriate is useful to the system and to future victims of OHCA.

MEASUREMENT OF PROFESSIONAL RESUSCITATION

Technological evolution in monitor/defibrillators has allowed collection of high fidelity data. Simultaneously, manufacturers have developed software to review, annotate, and understand these data. Some monitor/defibrillators also allow audio recording. The black box of OHCA is no longer. One can now understand and review moment by moment the actions of the crews as they cared for the patient. This insight can be a huge step forward for the individual trying to make change around his or her OHCA system of care.

Multiple examples exist of areas where the ability to review care has provided insight. One simple example is that of precharging the monitor/defibrillator prior to a pulse check. This process allows highly trained teams to minimize the perishock pause, where it is known that a short perishock pause is associated with increased survival from OHCA.[7]

Many EMS systems that have made strides in improving their survival from OHCA have found postincident review of monitor/defibrillator data to be a key and critical portion of their success. Providing feedback to the crews on the quality of their CPR, the number and length of their pauses, any delays in diagnosing arrhythmias, or other important findings can lead to significant team improvement in the future. This is a time-consuming endeavor, with review of a case anecdotally consuming between 30 and 60 minutes in the hands of an experienced reviewer and depending on the complexity of the resuscitation.

Systems that have implemented audio recordings, mandatory in King County, Washington, have found value in this technology. The ability provided by voice recording to understand why CPR was paused provides significant clarity over the more common situation of only acknowledging that the pause occurred and relying on recall when inquiring with the prehospital provider.

FIRST RESPONDER DEFIBRILLATION

Time and time again, early defibrillation has been found to dramatically impact survival from OHCA.[8] Most recently, using Resuscitation Outcomes Consortium data on 49,555 OHCA events, patients who received a shock from a bystander using an automated external defibrillator (AED) were significantly more likely to survive to discharge (66.5% vs 43.0%, $P<.001$).[9] EMTs have long been found to be competent and capable with AEDs in a rescue situation.[10] But is there an agency that can respond even before the fire first responders can arrive on scene? In many communities, police are distributed throughout a municipality and are constantly mobile throughout their assigned shift. The functional removal of turnout time (the time it takes fire and EMS to get to their rig and get the wheels rolling) significantly increases the probability of a successful defibrillatory effort. Extending first responder defibrillation to police is an idea that has logical appeal. It is not complicated, but it is not easy.

Equipping police agencies with AEDs and high-quality CPR training has been a successful strategy in many communities.[11,12] Police have generally been willing partners when approached.[13] Those communities most likely to benefit are suburban or rural, although some urban settings will benefit. Settings where EMS has a longer response time and police may be physically and temporally closer to the scene of an OHCA are more likely to see benefit from deployment of AEDs with police.

Obtaining buy-in from police is often more intricate. In some communities, the first AED defibrillation has been of a fellow officer who suffered an OHCA. These situations are of obvious value in establishing a program of active AED police response. Other characteristics of successful police AED response programs include programs that have active participation from the EMS and fire department sides of first response, police responders who are dispatched directly and specifically to an address rather than a radio broadcast like "AED needed".

Medical directors and leaders of EMS systems should integrate police in on the EMS response whenever possible. Making things simple for police first responders is a step that increases their participation level. Teaching hands-only CPR helps police with little medical training be able to competently treat OHCA in the interval before higher trained providers arrive on scene. Additionally, largely positive feedback should be provided. No officer is required to use his or her AED, but when he or she does, the praise is of a large volume and effusive.

Following these steps can help your locality develop and implement a police first response AED program. The more dispersed your community is, the longer your EMS response times, the more likely it is that police AED use will benefit an OHCA patient.

SMART TECHNOLOGIES FOR CARDIOPULMONARY RESUSCITATION/ AUTOMATED EXTERNAL DEFIBRILLATOR

How can technology aid the lay rescuer in OHCA? This question has been pondered the world over in a quest to increase survival. In the smartphone era, location data and connectivity are ubiquitous. Using these tools to link victims with rescuers will lead to a new era in the treatment of OHCA.

Several apps have emerged across the world that seek to extend the paradigm of calling for help that has been recommended to every CPR class attendee. The thought is that the voice can only travel so far; while professional rescuers can be activated quickly and have short response times in many cases, often a trained and capable provider might be right around the corner and yet unaware of the emergency unfolding nearby. Using digital connections from the dispatch center, willing volunteers can be activated through their smartphones to respond and provide care prior to arrival of the system-based first responders.

Further technology to link the location of nearby AEDs may lead to earlier defibrillation. Location information and registration of AEDs is one strategy to lead to their use in crisis scenarios. These AED registries, as they are often referred to, are tough to keep up to date, as AEDs and the entities that own them often relocate or reconfigure their space.

In a future state, it would be desirable for AEDs to be able to automatically report and update their location and status to a central repository that would be available to dispatchers and rescuers in times of need. The technology to do this exists today but is not yet commercially available.

CARDIOPULMONARY RESUSCITATION/ AUTOMATED EXTERNAL DEFIBRILLATOR TRAINING IN SCHOOLS

The first widely published call for CPR to be taught in schools came in the 2003 International Liaison Committee on Resuscitation consensus document.[14] The rationale here is that schools provide access to a large cross-section of the community. With sufficient time, training in schools will allow a large percentage of the community to be trained in CPR.

The American Heart Association recommended that this training occur in middle school or high school as students are likely to have enough size to effectively compress an adult thorax and are likely to retain their training.[15] Critical teaching points include recognition of an emergency, chest compressions as a psychomotor process and skills practice. AED awareness and training are also highly encouraged.

Several challenges exist in these training programs. The first is finding space in the existing curriculum to teach CPR and associated psychomotor skills. The second is that these classes often require outlay of financial resources for new equipment and curricula. These barriers are not insurmountable, and several states have solved them creatively including funding the training from the state department of education.

The impact of these programs is difficult to measure but predicted to be significant. At the very least, these programs increase familiarity with a skill that can be scary and intimidating to many lay persons. After training, students in high school have been shown to have a significant increase in positive emotions and a decrease in negative emotions around providing CPR.[16] As of this writing, 36 of the 50 states have mandated CPR training at some point prior to high school graduation.[17]

ACCOUNTABILITY TO COMMUNITY

Transparency has become paramount in governmental agencies and private organizations, and for good reason. Explaining the results an agency or organization has produced can be an effective way of communicating the work done and the value of that organization. Health care, and specifically EMS, has been behind the trend of other industries. Some large hospital systems have taken the lead on this issue. For example, Cleveland Clinic has been widely recognized for clearly reporting selected outcomes that greatly exceed those required by federal standards.[18] This clear and transparent accounting of quality allows the health care-consuming public to make informed decisions about scheduled medical care.

Transparency in EMS is more about demonstrating value and need. *Change occurs iteratively*, and through annual reporting, the progress of change in an organization can be clearly reported. One example of transparency and accountability to the community is the report issued annually to residents of King County, Washington (**Fig. 1**). This report details many aspects of the prehospital care the citizens of the county have received and benchmarks them against previous years. Other, similar strategies exist. The City of Seattle, Washington, for example, has a city government-wide Web site that lists, details, and creates trends for metrics from all aspects of government, including EMS (**Fig. 2**).

There are several important concepts to keep in mind when generating reports such as these. First, the metrics chosen for display should be easily understood and well explained. For example, listing a number and saying it is the cardiac arrest survival rate (eg, "45% survival rate") is disingenuous at best, and likely misleading. Instead, one should be careful to explain all the relevant nuances that go into standard Utstein reporting and how they are significant, at the layperson level. Secondly, when using newer media where data are regularly refreshable, caution is advised when setting the interval for updates. Updating a survival statistic with each cardiac arrest will lead to emotional swings in the EMS workforce that are unwarranted simply due to variation in patient presentation Instead, preselect an interval (eg, 3 or 6 months) that is appropriate for the size of community/number of worked cardiac arrests and then report data at that interval. This will lead to a smoothing of results that is, more accurate over the long term and better represents the work done by the agency.

The importance of clarity in writing and messaging cannot be overemphasized. These reports should and will be reviewed widely. They form the basis of support for the EMS organization in the community. They should be relevant and timely. Clarity and transparency will bring about accountability.

CULTURE OF EXCELLENCE

Caring for OHCA patients requires a team, tools, and an attitude. Defibrillator, box of medications, oxygen tank, backboard, metronome, and paramedic: which of these is most important to a successful resuscitation?

Several common elements are found in many high-performing systems with a culture of excellence. This first of these is an organizational vision that is clear, communicated, and understood by the people who make up the organization. This vision allows those who work in the organization to have a clear purpose and meaning. Organizations with a culture of excellence work to make all who participate in the system high performers. Those already performing at a high standard are celebrated, and those who are average performers are coached to improve.

Change in an organization can be extremely disruptive. In agencies with a culture of excellence, the motivation to achieve the vision of the organization is greater than the discomfort associated with the change itself. This single-minded way of moving forward through change helps those struggling with change to push through barriers, be they physical or mental.

Teams in an organization with a culture of excellence are highly collaborative. They work together

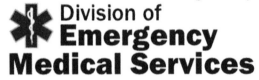

2017 Annual Report
to the King County Council
September 2017

Fig. 1. King County EMS Annual report: this report details the outcomes and processes for prehospital care in the county to provide transparency to the community. It is updated annually. (*From* Division of Emergency Medical Services. 2017 Annual Report to the King City Council. Public Health Seattle & King County 2017. p. 1. Available at: https://www.kingcounty.gov/depts/health/emergency-medical-services/reports.aspx. Accessed February 4, 2018; with permission.)

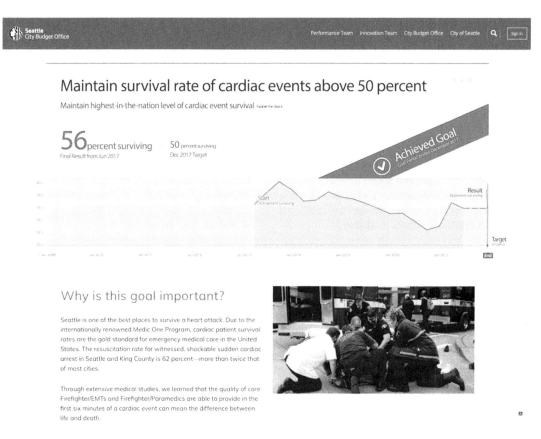

Fig. 2. Seattle outcomes reporting. This report updates the community on the progress of different metrics by the city government, including the fire department, which handles all EMS calls. Various metrics are measured and reported, and updated frequently throughout the year. A dynamic Web site allows for data to be updated more frequently, if appropriate for the data measure. (*From* Seattle City Budget Office, 2018. Public Safety. City of Seattle. Available at: https://performance.seattle.gov/stat/goals/wbgi-kcdb. Accessed February 5, 2018; with permission.)

well. Every member of the team has an eye toward the goal and does his or her part to move the objective forward. When the team succeeds, when the patient survives, everyone is responsible, and everyone feels satisfied.

Knowing those characteristics and assuming that they apply to EMS organizations as well, how can an organization establish a culture of excellence? Establishing a mindset of excellence is the first step. This is a shared mental model between all members of the organization around what excellence will look like. A good example in EMS organizations is the mantra *Everyone in VF Survives*. Once this mindset is shared, strategies to achieve this excellence can be disseminated. These can include skills and competencies that are required to achieve a state of excellence.

The most difficult step must then be undertaken. This step is sustainment. This is taking the new way and making it "the way things are done around here." Once change becomes permanent, a culture of excellence is truly in place.

Of all the items previously listed for a resuscitation, which is most important? As a culture of excellence develops, the backboard will become the most important tool at the scene of an OHCA. The backboard is most important, because the crew will start to bring it to the patient at the beginning of the case. Why bring it to the patient early? Because the crew will learn to expect the patient to survive. When the patient survives, you need to extricate them to the ambulance. The culture shift inherent in a mindset alteration to an expectation of survival is huge and will occur with hard work and implementation of a culture of excellence.

SUMMARY

The previously mentioned steps, while not the entirety of a successful, high-performing system of care for OHCA, will lead to significant gains for most, if not all, EMS systems. Many of the lessons translate well into hospital-based systems. As Dr

Eisenberg likes to say at the Resuscitation Academy, *If you have seen 1 EMS system, you have seen 1 EMS system*. This is especially true about OHCA care. Problems are local; solutions must be local as well. Lessons learned and best practices can inform decisions, but ultimately it is up to the medical direction and operations teams within an agency to get the work done.

For more information and related content, please refer to the Resuscitation Academy Web site at resuscitationacademy.org. Additionally, Dr. Eisenberg has authored a text ebook available on the Resuscitation Academy Web site with more detail on each of these steps as well as additional content. All content is freely available.

ACKNOWLEDGMENTS

The author would be remiss if those who forged the curriculum and lessons of the Resuscitation Academy and provided the knowledge and experience to relate these messages were not thanked. Mickey Eisenberg, Leonard Cobb, and Michael Copass were the foundation of the messages contained herein. Ann Doll, Peter Kudenchuk, Tom Rea, and Michael Sayre have carried this message on to new states, countries, and continents. The real-world practical knowledge passed on by Craig Aman, Mike Helbock, Jonathan Larson, and Norm Nedell is invaluable and informs the authors decisions as an EMS medical director every single day. Thank you all for your friendship, mentorship, and wonderful collegiality.

REFERENCES

1. Wu Z, Panczyk M, Spaite DW, et al. Telephone cardiopulmonary resuscitation is independently associated with improved survival and improved functional outcome after out-of-hospital cardiac arrest. Resuscitation 2018;122:135–40.

2. White L, Rogers J, Bloomingdale M, et al. Dispatcher-assisted cardiopulmonary resuscitation: risks for patients not in cardiac arrest. Circulation 2010;121(1):91–7.

3. American Heart Association. Telephone CPR (T-CPR) program recommendations and performance measures. 2018. Available at: http://cpr.heart.org/AHAECC/CPRAndECC/ResuscitationScience/TelephoneCPR/RecommendationsPerformanceMeasures/UCM_477526_Telephone-CPR-T-CPR-Program-Recommendations-and-Performance-Measures.jsp. Accessed January 27, 2018.

4. Fisk CA, Olsufka M, Yin L, et al. Lower-dose epinephrine administration and out-of-hospital cardiac arrest outcomes. Resuscitation 2018;124:43–8.

5. Harris AW, Kudenchuk PJ. Cardiopulmonary resuscitation: the science behind the hands. Heart 2018. https://doi.org/10.1136/heartjnl-2017-312696.

6. Nichol G, Cobb LA, Yin L, et al. Briefer activation time is associated with better outcomes after out-of-hospital cardiac arrest. Resuscitation 2016;107:139–44.

7. Cheskes S, Schmicker RH, Christenson J, et al. Perishock pause: an independent predictor of survival from out-of-hospital shockable cardiac arrest. Circulation 2011;124(1):58–66.

8. Weaver WD, Copass MK, Bufi D, et al. Improved neurologic recovery and survival after early defibrillation. Circulation 1984;69(5):943–8.

9. Pollack RA, Brown SP, Rea T, et al. Impact of bystander automated external defibrillator use on survival and functional outcomes in shockable observed public cardiac arrests. Circulation 2018. https://doi.org/10.1161/CIRCULATIONAHA.117.030700.

10. Eisenberg MS, Copass MK, Hallstrom AP, et al. Treatment of out-of-hospital cardiac arrests with rapid defibrillation by emergency medical technicians. N Engl J Med 1980;302(25):1379–83.

11. Becker L, Husain S, Kudenchuk P, et al. Treatment of cardiac arrest with rapid defibrillation by police in King County, Washington. Prehosp Emerg Care 2014;18(1):22–7.

12. Husain S, Eisenberg M. Police AED programs: a systematic review and meta-analysis. Resuscitation 2013;84(9):1184–91.

13. Aldeen AZ, Hartman ND, Segura A, et al. Video self-instruction for police officers in cardiopulmonary resuscitation and automated external defibrillators. Prehosp Disaster Med 2013;28(5):471–6.

14. Chamberlain DA, Hazinski MF. Education in resuscitation: an ILCOR symposium: Utstein Abbey: Stavanger, Norway: June 22-24, 2001. Circulation 2003;108(20):2575–94.

15. Cave DM, Aufderheide TP, Beeson J, et al. Importance and implementation of training in cardiopulmonary resuscitation and automated external defibrillation in schools: a science advisory from the American Heart Association. Circulation 2011;123(6):691–706.

16. Alismail A, Massey E, Song C, et al. Emotional impact of cardiopulmonary resuscitation training on high school students. Front Public Health 2017;5:362.

17. American Heart Association. CPR in schools legislation map. 2018. Available at: http://cpr.heart.org/AHAECC/CPRAndECC/Programs/CPRInSchools/UCM_475820_CPR-in-Schools-Legislation-Map.jsp. Accessed February 2, 2018.

18. Cleveland Clinic. Treatment outcomes. 2018. Available at: https://my.clevelandclinic.org/departments/clinical-transformation/depts/quality-patient-safety/treatment-outcomes. Accessed February 2, 2018.

The Critical Role of Dispatch

Saman Kashani, MD, MSc[a,b],*, Stephen Sanko, MD[a,b], Marc Eckstein, MD, MPH[a,b]

KEYWORDS

- Prehospital • Dispatch • Dispatcher • Public safety answering point • EMS • 9-1-1

KEY POINTS

- Call centers for 9-1-1 serve as de facto coordinating centers for emergency response in the United States.
- The roles of dispatch include information gathering, resource management, and provision of prearrival instructions.
- Prearrival instructions for cardiopulmonary resuscitation have been repeatedly demonstrated to enhance survival from out-of-hospital cardiac arrest.
- High performing systems are able to address common dispatching hurdles such as limited English proficiency callers, high-volume days, disaster management, and the increasing volume of low-acuity callers.

 Audio content accompanies this article at http://www.cardiology.theclinics.com.

Dispatcher—"9-1-1, what is your emergency?"
Caller—"My grandmother just passed out! Please send help!"
Dispatcher—"I show you calling from XXX-XXXX, is that correct?"
Caller—"Please send help, are you coming? She's turning blue!"

Every year in the United States, 9-1-1 is activated 240 million times across 5806 primary and secondary public safety answering point (PSAPs), more commonly referred to as dispatch centers.[1] The 9-1-1 system is relatively young, but the role of the emergency medical dispatcher (EMD) and the 9-1-1 system as a whole has developed significantly since its beginning. It provides thousands of communities with an umbrella of security—help is only a phone call away.

Emergency dispatch is the use of a professional telecommunicator to gather information, assign resources, and coordinate layperson and emergency responders in the prehospital setting. It plays a critical role in day-to-day emergency response for local police, fire, and emergency medical services (EMS), resource allocation, disaster response, and public health and acts as the de facto coordination center of many jurisdictions. The importance of the emergency dispatch system and the sense of security that it provides to the community cannot be overstated. High-performance 9-1-1 call centers strive for prompt call answering, low call-processing times for time-critical emergencies, efficient initial dispatch of the most appropriate EMS resource(s), and successful recruitment of bystanders into performing life-saving interventions prior to EMS arrival.

Disclosure: The authors have nothing to disclose.
a Los Angeles Fire Department, EMS Bureau, 200 North Main Street, Suite 1860, Los Angeles, CA 90012, USA;
b Division of Emergency Medical Services, Department of Emergency Medicine, Keck School of Medicine of USC, 1200 North State Street, Room 1011, Los Angeles, CA 90033, USA
* Corresponding author. Department of Emergency Medicine, Keck School of Medicine of the University of Southern California, 1200 North State Street, Room 1011, Los Angeles, CA 90033-1029.
E-mail address: saman.kashani@med.usc.edu

Cardiol Clin 36 (2018) 343–350
https://doi.org/10.1016/j.ccl.2018.03.001
0733-8651/18/© 2018 Elsevier Inc. All rights reserved.

EMS is a locally driven institution. Protocols and policies can vary widely depending on resource availability, population dynamics, and community needs. What follows is a general description of the history, operations, and critical value to patients of high-performance 9-1-1 dispatch, although there is considerable regional variability.

HISTORY OF EMERGENCY MEDICAL SERVICES IN THE UNITED STATES

The need for an organized response to medical emergencies was brought to the forefront when the National Academy of Sciences released "Accidental Death and Disability: The Neglected Disease of Modern Society" in 1966.[2] This landmark report identified the inadequacy of prehospital care at the time and its contribution to morbidity and mortality. This was followed shortly after by the era of modern emergency medical dispatch in the early 1970s, where the ability to send appropriate resources to a patient and provide emergency instructions to a caller prior to arrival of first responders were identified as an important link in the chain of survival.[3] This continues today, where the American Heart Association (AHA) identifies activation of EMS as the first link in the out-of-hospital cardiac arrest (OHCA) chain of survival.[4]

The first national effort to support EMS as a profession was through the Emergency Medical Service Systems Act of 1973 and creation of the National Registry of Emergency Medical Technicians, which led to the development of the emergency medical technician (EMT) and EMT-paramedic designation in the early to mid-1970s. The first reported use of emergency medical dispatch occurred in Phoenix, Arizona, in 1975. There, a paramedic gave telephone instructions to the mother of an apneic child. The child survived and since then many systems across the world have begun to provide emergency instructions to callers before emergency responders arrive.[5] In Washington State in 1982, University of Washington Professor Mickey Eisenberg began training 9-1-1 dispatchers to provide instructions to layperson callers on how to perform cardiopulmonary resuscitation (CPR) over the phone. These were the earliest iterations of prearrival instructions (PAIs).

PRIMARY AND SECONDARY PUBLIC SAFETY ANSWERING POINTS

Centers that receive 9-1-1 telephone calls are referred to as PSAPs, or more commonly dispatch centers. The 9-1-1 number was created in the late 1970s through the efforts of the Federal Communications Commission and AT&T. It was eventually adopted as a universal emergency phone number for all police, fire, and medical emergencies.[6] Depending on the needs of the community, there may be a single combined PSAP for all types of emergencies or each emergency response agency may have their own.

THE COMPONENTS OF AN EMERGENCY MEDICAL SERVICES DISPATCH SYSTEM

As the chain of survival suggests, there are multiple factors involved in successfully resuscitating a patient in the field. To understand the vital role of dispatch, it helps to understand the available resources and the 9-1-1 dispatch response mechanism (**Fig. 1**). For example, one of the roles of the dispatcher is allocating the "right resources for the right patient." Similar to the in-hospital setting, there is a spectrum of potential prehospital care providers that might respond to an emergency.

First is the caller or bystanders who activate 9-1-1. They begin the chain reaction that leads to definitive care.

Callers have traditionally been separated into 4 types[7]:

- A first-party caller is the patient.
- A second-party caller is a person within proximity of the patient who can potentially provide care to the patient.
- A third-party caller is not within proximity of the patient (eg, motorist driving by an accident).
- A fourth-party caller is another public service agency or dispatch (eg, law enforcement or airport dispatch).

Until EMS can arrive on scene, time-critical interventions like CPR and defibrillation can be performed by layperson responders who have either been previously trained in first aid or who can be trained in real time through PAIs provided by the dispatcher.[8] One way of bridging the gap until professional rescuers arrive is converting third-party callers to a second-party callers so that they are in a position to receive and act on PAIs.

Description of all types of professional rescuers is outside the scope of this article, but it is important to have a rudimentary understanding of the EMS system in a jurisdiction. Skill level can vary greatly by type of rescuer and even among rescuers of the same level in different jurisdictions. For example, a paramedic in one jurisdiction may be authorized to intubate children whereas a paramedic in another jurisdiction may not. Regional variability is based on local protocols, population needs, medical oversight, equipment, and training.[9] **Table 1** provides a description of common EMS providers and their associated scope of practice.

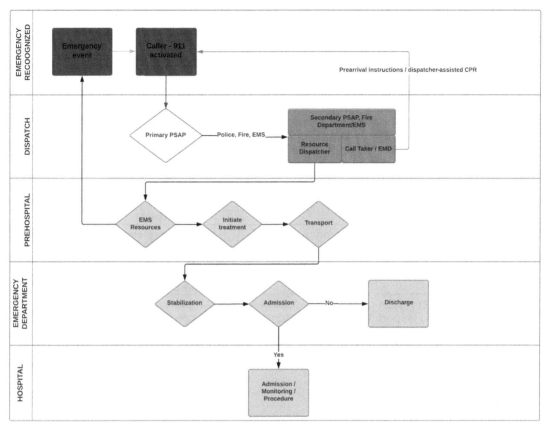

Fig. 1. Typical 9-1-1 call processing begins with the recognition of an emergency leading to a 9-1-1 call. The call is taken at the primary PSAP, which in many cases is a service of the local law enforcement agency. If medically related, the call may be handed off to a secondary PSAP where the call taker, if trained in emergency medical dispatch, can provide PAIs like CPR to the caller. Concurrently, a resource dispatcher is coordinating the activation of field resources, like ambulances, which can then treat and transport the patient. A general description of 9-1-1 call processing is provided; each jurisdiction may differ in the agency and staffing of their dispatch center.

THE MULTIPLE ROLES OF DISPATCH

From the moment 9-1-1 is activated, dispatch choreographs multiple activities, including information gathering, resource management, and provision of PAIs. Both the AHA and the European Resuscitation Council identified the dispatcher role in 2015 as a crucial part of OHCA survival.[11,12]

First and foremost, the EMD is an information gatherer. The most fundamental role of the 9-1-1 call taker is to establish the location of the incident and obtain a callback number. This simple-sounding task can be exceedingly complicated when the number of limited-English proficiency callers, callers unwilling to provide callback phone numbers, and callers who cannot recall critical information or are otherwise too emotional are taken into account. Although some jurisdictions have automatic number identification and automatic location identification, others do not. Even in jurisdictions with automatic number identification/automatic location identification systems, number

recognition often depends on a caller using a landline phone number. Between 1994 and 2014, the number of US mobile phone subscriptions increased from 9.1 per 100 people to 110.2 per 100 people and with it 9-1-1 calls from cellular devices.[1,13] Even when a general location is identified, obtaining enough information to guide emergency responders can be complicated. For example, a 9-1-1 cell phone call originating at an airport, mall, college campus, high-rise, parking garage, or outdoor park poses unique challenges for an EMD in pinpointing the exact location of the patient. A common misconception is that a dispatcher can see an exact location based on a cell phone's GPS signal. Although efforts are being made toward this goal, it is far from universally available or reliable. Ultimately, most dispatch systems rely on the caller to provide an exact location or must rely on the location of the nearest cell site.

The next role of the dispatcher is as a resource manager. Based on the information gathered, or

Table 1
Emergency medical services providers

Title	Description	Examples of Scope of Practice[a]
Prehospital		
First responder	Umbrella term for any person who responds initially to an emergency Can be nonmedical personnel (eg, law enforcement officer). The term is not a reference to scope of practice but rather arrival to the scene.	Variable
Emergency medical responder[10]	Basic medical training focused on lifesaving interventions; not the primary care giver	Supplemental oxygen, repositioning the airway, bag-valve-mask ventilation, automated external defibrillator
EMT basic[10]	Basic skills focused on the acute management and transportation	Commonly referred to as basic life support skills; includes emergency medical responder skills plus assist in medication delivery, and patient transport
Advanced EMT[10] • Previously EMT intermediate	Combination of advanced and basic life support. In some rural settings may be the most advanced prehospital emergency responder	EMT-basic skills plus intravenous access, supraglottic airways, limited pharmacologic interventions
EMT paramedic[10]	Invasive emergency medical treatment Advanced life support	Advanced EMT skills plus intubation, advanced cardiac life support, needle thoracostomy, defibrillation, and cardioversion
EMS advanced provider	Nurse practitioner or physician assistant	Parenteral medications, suturing, point-of-care testing
PSAP		
9-1-1 Call taker/ emergency dispatcher	Professional telecommunicator; may not have medical training (eg, police or firefighter dispatchers)	
EMD	Professional telecommunicator who is certified as an EMD, which includes training in providing PAIs	
Hospital		
Mobile intensive care nurse	Generally, emergency department nurse with additional training to provide online medical control to EMS personnel	
Base hospital physician	Generally, an emergency medicine–trained physician who is familiar with prehospital care and can provide an added level of online medical control	
EMS physician	Emergency medicine trained physician with subspecialty training in EMS system design, policy, procedure, and management; may be subspecialty board certified in EMS	

[a] Not comprehensive. Scope of practice varies by region.

at times the limited information, the dispatcher selects a dispatch code, which is preprogrammed for a particular dispatch algorithm. One size does not fill all. This is often referred to as the maximal response dilemma. Like hospital resources, there are a finite number of emergency responders. Imagine if multiple EMS vehicles were sent lights and sirens to all 240 million 9-1-1 calls per year. The impact on traffic patterns, increased risk of motor vehicle accidents, and rapid exhaustion of emergency resources would be catastrophic.[3] Many systems use the 8-minute standard to respond to all 9-1-1 calls regardless of their complexity or acuity.[14,15] Dispatching a system's resources unnecessarily, in particular, is of great concern because if, for example, a paramedic unit is dispatched to a basic life support call, then it is not available for a time-critical call like a witnessed cardiac arrest, where the patient may benefit from advanced life support skills and rapid arrival.[15,16] Based on a call's needs, the most appropriate resources should be sent to the call. Although some dispatch systems send "everyone to everything," most high-volume systems use some component of tiered dispatching. This conserves resources for the next call by only sending the minimum number of resources to any particular call.

Lastly, provision of telephonic emergency instructions or PAIs is a dispatcher's next role. This requires additional certification to the level of EMD but has been recognized as a crucial function of a PSAP by the National Association of EMS Physicians and is an expectation of many communities.[17]

Chief among these are instructions for CPR in OHCA. These patients, in particular, have little chance of meaningful survival unless early cases of cardiac arrest are recognized by an EMD and high-quality CPR is initiated by bystanders.[18] PAIs are meant to maximize the chance of survival until emergency responders can arrive, and emergency priority dispatch systems are the set of protocols adopted by various PSAPs to help EMDs provide medical care. Earliest among these systems was the Medical Priority Dispatch System, created by Dr Jeff Clawson. Other systems have developed since then, such as the Association of Public-Safety Communications Officials International; the Criteria Based Dispatch in Seattle, Washington; and the Los Angeles Tiered Dispatch System.[19,20] All these systems focus on logic-driven, scripted questions to interrogate callers, identify appropriate resources for dispatch, and provide emergency instructions (**Fig. 2**).

DISPATCHER-ASSISTED CARDIOPULMONARY RESUSCITATION

Early recognition of cardiac arrest and initiation of dispatcher-assisted CPR (DA-CPR) is fundamental to successful resuscitation. Not only does it promote early bystander CPR but also is itself associated with increased survival.[18] The EMD systems, described previously, use scripted questions to increase the likelihood of identifying OHCA. The 2015 AHA guidelines stress the importance of assessing consciousness and breathing through scripted questions, such as the ones used by Los Angeles Tiered Dispatch System and Seattle Criteria Based Dispatch that ask callers, "Are they awake" followed by "Are they breathing *normally*."[21] Scripted questions are designed to move the caller within proximity of the patient and avoid time-consuming and inaccurate activities like counting respirations or pulse rate. It also has good specificity to recognize cardiac arrest.[22–24] If the answer to these questions is no or is unclear, the dispatcher then immediately provides CPR emergency instructions (Audio 1). Agonal breathing, in particular, is important for the EMD to identify because it has been associated with 50% of unrecognized cardiac arrests.[25] Early recognition of inadequate breathing is crucial to prompting layperson resuscitation and improving neurologic outcomes (Audio 1).[26]

BARRIERS TO DISPATCHER-ASSISTED CARDIOPULMONARY RESUSCITATION

Recognition of cardiac arrest and inadequate breathing is difficult even in a hospital setting.[12,27] Obtaining this information from a layperson caller is even more complicated although not impossible. Challenges include callers with limited English proficiency, emotional or hysterical callers, and those who are unwilling to initiate CPR out of fear of harming the patient or themselves. Elderly or very young callers may not be able to physically position the patient appropriately. Overall, fewer than 6% of patients with OHCA survive to hospital discharge but some communities have survival rates closer to 60%.[28] What this reveals is that these barriers are not insurmountable but rather engaging the caller in a way to elicit information and then converting that information into action is possible through adjustments in policy, community outreach, and education, one example of which was the AHA formal recommendation of chest compression–only DA-CPR in 2017.[29]

HIGH-VOLUME DAYS, DISASTER MANAGEMENT, AND OTHER TIME-CRITICAL SCENARIOS

Most literature and dispatcher metrics focus on OHCA. Busy 9-1-1 call takers, however, frequently find themselves guiding callers and patients through other complex time-critical scenarios. Whether the call is a multivehicle car accident or an apneic child, a dispatcher's job is highly complex and requires the ability to quickly jump

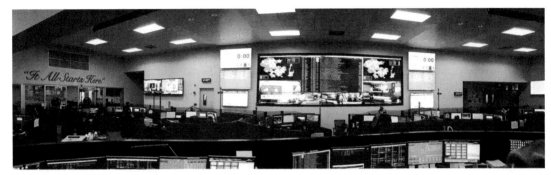

Fig. 2. Los Angeles Fire Department Metropolitan Fire Communications. Dispatch centers are designed to provide maximum situational awareness to the prehospital providers.

between different emergency protocols while maintaining dispatcher-caller rapport. Furthermore, protocols may vary depending on system status and the nature of the emergency (eg, resource allocation and PAIs during a surge event, such as an earthquake or wildland fire). These types of events often require the dispatcher to work in a degraded mode where fewer than typical resources or no resources are dispatched. Scenarios like these reinforce that the efforts of well-trained telecommunicators are critically important to 9-1-1 systems.

CALL TAKER RESILIENCE

Like their hospital and prehospital colleagues, 9-1-1 call takers are faced with very stressful situations. Unlike their colleagues, however, they frequently are not made aware of a patient's ultimate diagnosis or outcome and have the added stress of managing emergencies without seeing the patient. This is quite stressful, and rates of depression are of concern. Dispatcher stress can be objectively measured through cortisol levels, and persistently elevated stress levels are detrimental to long-term health outcomes.[30,31] An increasing number of prank calls, calling to talk when lonely, or calling for nonemergencies (eg, paying parking tickets) add to an already overburdened system by not only saturating emergency lines but also fatiguing finite and valuable call taker resources. There is a great need for further studies in providing constructive feedback, performance improvement, and promotion of dispatcher resilience.

LOW-ACUITY CALLERS

Low-acuity patients are increasingly using the 9-1-1 system. Medicare data from 2005 to 2009 indicate that up to 13% to 16% of EMS transports were nonemergent or primary care related, whereas another 34% of patients treated in an emergency department had low-acuity diagnosis.[32] The impact

of non-emergent calls is an additional burden on EMS systems at a time when call volume is increasing across all call types.[33] Many of these callers access 9-1-1 because of barriers to traditional health care, such as limited English language proficiency, social or mental health barriers, and mobility restrictions.[32–36] To ensure that the finite 9-1-1 resources are available for time-critical calls, such as cardiac arrest or respiratory distress, PSAPs having been instituting low-acuity protocols that send fewer or no resources to nonemergent callers.[37] Instead, these callers are referred to alternate locations like a clinic or local hospital. In recent years, some PSAPs have leveraged the increased diagnostic skills of nurses and other providers for low-acuity calls that have been screened by 9-1-1 call takers to improve patient triage and navigation.[38–40]

FUTURE OF 9-1-1 DISPATCH

Systems for 9-1-1 are under pressure to keep pace with modern technology. A majority of 9-1-1 systems throughout the country, however, were created using analog systems intended to carry voice information alone. Of the 240 million 9-1-1 calls, an estimated 80% originate from mobile devices and, when comparing 2014 and 2015 data, cellular phone usage increased by 31%, Voice over Internet Protocol usage increased by 78%, multiline telephone systems increased by 127%, and text–to–9-1-1 usage increased by 3442%.[41] Moving forward, dispatch centers need to keep pace with the technology in the hands of the public. There are multiple national efforts toward this goal. Enhanced 9-1-1 is already available in most of areas covered by 9-1-1 and indicates the system's ability to approximately automatically locate the caller and direct the call to the most geographically appropriate PSAP. It also allows for limited transmission of data elements like text messages.[42]

Next-generation 9-1-1 (NG9-1-1) takes this one step further by restructuring the existing narrow-band 9-1-1 system into a more modern digital Internet protocol–based system that would not only use GPS to locate the precise location of the caller but also allow for transmission of text or video while providing for greater interoperability between emergency service providers. NG9-1-1 promises to make PSAPs more proactive rather than reactive. For example, using NG9-1-1 technology, a dispatcher may leverage the more accurate location of an emergency caller and send out alerts to nearby layperson first responders or let the victims of a multicar traffic collision know that help is on the way.

SUMMARY

Emergency medical dispatch has evolved over the years. Strong dispatch systems contribute to and strengthen the early links in the chain of care of OHCA. Timely recognition of an emergency, early CPR, and PAIs as well as the efficient allocation of prehospital resources are vital.

SUPPLEMENTARY DATA

Supplementary data related to this article can be found online at https://doi.org/10.1016/j.ccl.2018.03.001.

REFERENCES

1. National Emergency Number Association: the 911 Association. 2017. Available at: www.nena.org. Accessed October 20, 2017.
2. Cowley RA. Accidental death and disability: the neglected disease of modern society - where is the fifth component? Ann Emerg Med 1982;11(10):576–81.
3. Clawson JJ. EMS dispatch. In: Cone DC, editor. Emergency medical services: clinical practice and systems oversight. 2nd edition. Indianapolis (IN): Priority Press; 2015. p. 94–112.
4. American Heart Association. Web-based integrated guidelines for cardiopulmonary resuscitation and emergency cardiovascular care – part 4: systems of care and continuous quality improvement. ECC-guidelines.heart.org. 2015:2–3.
5. Zachariah BS, Medical S. The development of emergency medical dispatch in the USA: a historical perspective. Eur J Emerg Med 1995;2(3):1979–82.
6. 9-1-1 Origin & History. NENA The 9-1-1 Association. Available at: http://www.nena.org/?page=911 overviewfacts. Accessed December 14, 2017.
7. Clawson JJ, Sinclair R. The emotional content and cooperation score in emergency medical dispatching. Prehosp Emerg Care 2001;5(1):29–35.
8. Roppolo LP, Pepe PE, Cimon N, et al. Modified cardiopulmonary resuscitation (CPR) instruction protocols for emergency medical dispatchers: rationale and recommendations. Resuscitation 2005;65(2):203–10.
9. Williams I, Valderrama AL, Bolton P, et al. Factors associated with emergency medical services scope of practice for acute cardiovascular events. Prehosp Emerg Care 2012;16(2):189–97.
10. The National Highway Traffic Safety Administration. The National EMS scope of practice model. Washington, DC: National Highway Traffic Safety Administration; 2005.
11. Neumar RW, Shuster M, Callaway CW, et al. Part 1: executive summary: 2015 American Heart Association guidelines update for cardiopulmonary resuscitation and emergency cardiovascular care. Circulation 2015;132. https://doi.org/10.1161/CIR.0000000000000252.
12. Greif R, Lockey AS, Conghan P, et al. European resuscitation council guidelines for resuscitation 2015 section 10. Education and implementation of resuscitation. Resuscitation 2015;95:288–301.
13. CTIA. Getting 9-1-1 Location Accuracy Right. Available at: https://www.ctia.org/industry-data/facts-and-infographics-details/fact-and-infographics/getting-9-1-1-location-accuracy-right. Accessed January 1, 2018.
14. NFPA. National Fire Protection Association 1710 Standard for the Organization and Deployment of Fire Suppression Operations, Emergency Operations and Special Operations to the Public by Career Fire Departments. 2016.
15. Eisenberg MS, Bergner L, Hallstrom AP. Cardiac resuscitation in the community: importance of rapid provision and implications for program planning. JAMA 1979;241(18):1905–7.
16. Pell JP, Sirel JM, Marsden AK, et al. Effect of reducing ambulance response times on deaths from out of hospital cardiac arrest: cohort study. BMJ 2001;322(7299):1385–8.
17. NAEMSP. Emergency medical dispatch: position statement. Prehosp Emerg Care 2008;12(2):217.
18. Rea TD, Eisenberg MS, Culley LL, et al. Dispatcher-assisted cardiopulmonary resuscitation and survival in cardiac arrest. Circulation 2001;104(21):2513–6.
19. Culley L, Henwood D, Clark J, et al. Increasing the efficiency of emergency medical services by using criteria based dispatch. Ann Emerg Med 1994;24(5):867–72.
20. Sanko S, Lane C, Flinders A, et al. Impact of a new medical dispatch system on telecommunicator-assisted CPR. Ann Emerg Med 2016;68:S7.
21. Kronick SL, Kurz MC, Lin S, et al. Part 4: systems of care and continuous quality improvement: 2015 American Heart Association guidelines update for cardiopulmonary resuscitation and emergency cardiovascular care. Circulation 2015;132(18):S397–413.

22. Culley LL, Clark JJ, Eisenberg MS, et al. Dispatcher-assisted telephone CPR: common delays and time standards for delivery. Ann Emerg Med 1991;20(4): 362–6.

23. Clark JJ, Pat Larsen M, Culley LL, et al. Incidence of agonal respirations in sudden cardiac arrest. Ann Emerg Med 1992;21:1464–7.

24. Perkins GD, Walker G, Christensen K, et al. Teaching recognition of agonal breathing improves accuracy of diagnosing cardiac arrest teaching recognition of agonal breathing. Resuscitation 2006;70:432–7.

25. Vaillancourt C, Verma A, Trickett J, et al. Evaluating the effectiveness of dispatch-assisted cardiopulmonary resuscitation instructions. Acad Emerg Med 2007;14(10):877–83.

26. Cummins R, Ornato J, Thies W, et al. Improving survival from sudden cardiac arrest: the "chain of survival" concept. A statement for health professionals from the Advanced Cardiac Life Support Subcommittee and the Emergency Cardiac Care Committee, American Heart Association. Circulation 1991;83: 1832–47.

27. Smereka J, Szarpak Ł, Czyzewski Ł, et al. Are physicians able to recognition ineffective (agonal) breathing as element of cardiac arrest? Am J Emerg Med 2016;34:1165.

28. Graham R, Mccoy MA, Schultz AM. Strategies to improve cardiac arrest survival: a time to act. Committee on the treatment of cardiac arrest: current status and future directions; board on health sciences policy; institute of medicine. Washington, DC: National Academies Press; 2015.

29. Kleinman ME, Goldberger ZD, Rea T, et al. 2017 American Heart Association focused update on adult basic life support and cardiopulmonary resuscitation quality: an update to the American Heart Association guidelines for cardio pulmonary resuscitation and emergency cardiovascular care. Circulation 2017. https://doi.org/10.1161/CIR.0000000000000539.

30. Sapolsky RM. Why stress is bad for your brain. Science 1996;7(273):749–50.

31. Weibel L, Gabrion I, Aussedat M, et al. Work-related stress in an emergency medical dispatch center. Ann Emerg Med 2003;41(4):500–6.

32. Alpert A, Morganti KG, Margolis GS, et al. Giving EMS flexibility in transporting low-acuity patients could generate substantial Medicare savings. Health Aff (Millwood) 2013;32(12):2142–8.

33. Munjal KG, Silverman RA, Freese J, et al. Utilization of emergency medical services in a large urban area: description of call types and temporal trends. Prehosp Emerg Care 2011;15(3):371–80.

34. Scott J, Strickland AP, Warner K, et al. Frequent callers to and users of emergency medical systems: a systematic review. Emerg Med J 2014;31(8):684–91.

35. Kashani S, Ito T, Guggenheim A, et al. Implementation of a nurse practitioner response unit in an urban EMS system. Ann Emerg Med 2016;68(4 Supplement 1):S37.

36. Larkin GL, Claassen CA, Pelletier AJ, et al. National study of ambulance transports to United States emergency departments: importance of mental health problems. Prehosp Disaster Med 2006; 21(2):82–90.

37. Clawson JJ, Dernocoeur KB. Determinant codes versus response exerpts from: the principles of emergency medical dispatch. 3rd edition. Springville (UT): Liberty Press; 2009.

38. Krumperman K, Weiss S, Fullerton L, et al. Commentary on "two types of prehospital systems interventions that triage low-acuity patients to alternative sites of care". South Med J 2015;108(7). https://doi.org/10.14423/SMJ.0000000000000303.

39. Infinger A, Studnek JR, Hawkins E, et al. Implementation of prehospital dispatch protocols that triage low-acuity patients to advice-line nurses. Prehosp Emerg Care 2013;17(4):481–5.

40. Schmidt T, Neely KW, Adams AL, et al. Is it possible to safely triage callers to EMS dispatch centers to alternative resources? Prehosp Emerg Care 2003; 7(3):368–74.

41. National 911 Program. 2016 National 911 Progress Report. US Department of Transportation. National Highway Traffic Safety Administration; 2016.

42. Nguyen A. You can now text an emergency message to 911 in Los Angeles County. Los Angeles Times 2017.

Cardiopulmonary Resuscitation Quality Issues

Essie Reed-Schrader, MD[a], William T. Rivers, MD[a],
Lynn J. White, MS[b], Brian M. Clemency, DO[a],*

KEYWORDS

- Cardiac arrest • Cardiopulmonary resuscitation • Out-of-hospital cardiac arrest
- Emergency medical services • Heart massage

KEY POINTS

- Much of the current evidence and many of the recent treatment recommendations for increasing survival from cardiac arrest revolve around improving the quality of cardiopulmonary resuscitation during resuscitation.
- A focus on providing treatments that are proved beneficial and providing these treatments reliably, using measurement, monitoring, and implementation of quality-improvement strategies, will help to eliminate variation in outcomes and provide a foundation from which future improvements in resuscitation care can be developed.
- Using the knowledge and tools available today will help reduce the ambiguity and variability that exists in resuscitation today and provide the ability to save more lives in communities.

High-quality cardiopulmonary resuscitation (CPR) and defibrillation, if indicated, are the central interventions in the initial resuscitation from sudden cardiac arrest (SCA). Chest compressions, however, are often given either too slow or too fast or include inappropriate pressure on the chest during relaxation. Prolonged interruptions in compressions are frequent during resuscitation attempts.[1] Poor-quality CPR, with prolonged pauses for any cause, is associated with worse outcomes.[2] When external chest compressions and appropriate ventilation are provided effectively after collapse, it is possible to extend the prehospital treatment window for victims of SCA.[3]

The importance of providing high-quality compressions was not widely appreciated by either prehospital or hospital providers until the late 1990s. Treatment guidelines in the 1990s resulted in long pauses for ventilation and added lengthy interruptions in compressions to allow for performance of intubation, stacked shocks with frequent pulse checks, and medication administration. Emphasis on these treatments conveyed the perception that compressions were much less important than these other therapies.

It is now understood that poor compression quality can significantly affect perfusion and contributes to poor outcome.[2,4] With that realization and with a renewed focus on training to provide high-quality compressions, there is a growing awareness of the need to refocus on basic resuscitation components using strategies known to improve outcomes, particularly improving the quality of CPR, and the importance of having a well-coordinated system

Disclosure Statement: The authors have nothing to disclose.
[a] Department of Emergency Medicine, University at Buffalo, 462 Grider Street, Buffalo, NY 14215, USA;
[b] American Medical Response, 6363 S. Fiddlers Green Cir., Greenwood Village, CO 80111, USA
* Corresponding author.
E-mail address: bc34@buffalo.edu

Cardiol Clin 36 (2018) 351–356
https://doi.org/10.1016/j.ccl.2018.03.002
0733-8651/18/© 2018 Elsevier Inc. All rights reserved.

of care in a community.[5] This article reviews current evidence, recommendations, and best practices related to prehospital CPR quality.

CURRENT EVIDENCE

Current evidence regarding the effectiveness of CPR strategies is summarized by the International Liaison Committee on Resuscitation (ILCOR) in the form of their Treatment Recommendations (CoSTR).[6] These treatment recommendations form the basis of the guidelines disseminated by each of the ILCOR council members, including the American Heart Association (AHA), whose guidelines are consulted throughout North America. Recently, ILCOR has moved from holding a focused evidence review every 5 years to instituting a continuous evidence review and evaluating key resuscitation questions as evidence becomes available.

One of the limitations of treatment recommendations and subsequent guidelines arises from the low quality of available evidence for many advanced life support (ALS) treatments. Because there is a belief that clear guidelines are needed, many ALS treatment recommendations with low or very low evidence are strengthened by consensus of the experts and recommendations currently active are not changed without sufficient supporting evidence.

INTERNATIONAL LIAISON COMMITTEE ON RESUSCITATION TREATMENT RECOMMENDATIONS PERTINENT TO CARDIOPULMONARY RESUSCITATION QUALITY
Compression Rate

Chest compression rates have been shown to correlate with return of spontaneous circulation (ROSC), survival to discharge, and survival with favorable neurologic outcomes.[7] The recommended rate for compressions has increased since the initial version of the CPR guidelines, which were published in 1960 and recommended a rate of 60 compressions/min.[8] The 2010 AHA guidelines called for a rate of at least 100 compressions/min without specifying an upper limit.[4] Studies suggest that there is no benefit with regard to either ROSC or survival to discharge, when compressions are provided at the upper limit of 140 per minute.[8] The 2015 AHA guidelines reflect this evidence, stating that "it is reasonable" for compressions to be performed at a rate of 100 compressions/min to 120 compressions/min.[3] The ILCOR CoSTR recommendation states:

- We recommend a manual chest compression rate of 100 to 120/min (strong recommendation, very-low-quality evidence).[9]

Inappropriately fast compression rates may have deleterious effects due to inadequate time for filling of the heart between compressions and provider fatigue.[10,11]

Delivery of Chest Compressions

Several strategies have been proposed to attempt to optimize perfusion and/or to minimize/manipulate pauses during chest compressions. These methods include the provision of continuous compressions with asynchronous ventilation,[12] which showed no statistically significant difference in outcome when compared with conventional CPR. Another method is called minimally interrupted cardiac resuscitation (MICR), one strategy of which is called cardiocerebral resuscitation,[13] which consists of an initial series of cycles of uninterrupted chest compressions, passive ventilation, and before-and-after rhythm analysis with shock if appropriate. This cardiocerebral resuscitation strategy was studied in a large before and after trial comparing survival to hospital discharge in patients receiving standard advanced cardiac life support care versus those receiving minimally interrupted chest compressions in the prehospital setting. Survival to hospital discharge increased from 1.8% before MICR to 5.4% after MICR implementation.[13] Although this is an impressive improvement, it is unclear whether such a strategy would provide a similar effect in a system that had already had a survival rate at or above the Cardiac Arrest Registry to Enhance Survival (CARES) average of 10.8%.[14]

The newest of these delivery strategies currently being studied in an animal laboratory is a form of variable-rate CPR, sometimes referred to as stutter CPR.[15] This form of experimental CPR delivery is based on the concept of controlling pauses during CPR to invoke ischemic preconditioning mechanisms after SCA.

The 2015 treatment recommendations for chest compression from ILCOR include the following:

- EMS providers should perform CPR with 30 compressions to 2 ventilations or continuous chest compression with positive pressure ventilation delivered without pausing chest compressions until a tracheal tube or supraglottic device has been placed (strong recommendation, high-quality evidence).[9]
- For EMS systems that have adopted MICR, this strategy is considered a reasonable alternative

to conventional CPR for witnessed shockable out-of-hospital cardiac arrest (weak recommendation, very-low-quality evidence).[9]

Compression Depth

Guidelines for a precise depth of adult compressions were first introduced by the AHA in 2005 at approximately 4 cm to 5 cm[16] and were slightly revised in 2015 to at least 5 cm while allowing complete chest recoil after each compression.[4] After the 2010 recommendations, Vadeboncoeur and colleagues[17] demonstrated a positive association between compression depth and survival from prehospital cardiac arrest. It was also shown, however, that compression depths greater than 5.1 cm were associated with a decrease in survival with good neurologic outcomes. Similarly, Stiell and colleagues[18] demonstrated that the rate of survival increased as the chest compression depth increased; however, the benefit seemed to fall off at the extreme ends of depth (>5.0 cm), with the highest rates of survival to discharge occurring in the range of 4.0 cm to 5.5 cm. Based in part on these findings, the most recent guidelines call for a compression depth of "at least 5 cm for an average adult, while avoiding excessive chest compression depths greater than 6 cm."[9] The ILCOR treatment recommendations state:

- We recommend a chest compression depth of approximately 5 cm (2 in.) (strong recommendation, low-quality evidence) while avoiding excessive chest compression depths (greater than 6 cm [>2.4 in.] in an average adult) (weak recommendation, low-quality evidence) during manual CPR.[9]

Multiple studies have shown that chest compressions are often delivered with inadequate depth.[17,18]

Ventilation

Ventilations are recommended at a rate of 2 breaths every 30 compressions or 12 breaths to 15 breaths/min. The 30:2 compression to ventilation pattern has been shown superior to a 15:2 and to have similar outcomes as the strategy of providing asynchronous ventilations with continuous chest compressions in adult patients.[19] Despite the 30:2 recommendation, hyperventilation is common and may lead to increased intrathoracic pressure.[20] This increased intrathoracic pressure has been shown to reduce coronary perfusion pressure and rates of survival in animal models.[21,22] The ILCOR treatment recommendations state:

- We suggest a compression–ventilation ratio of 30:2 compared with any other compression–ventilation ratio in patients in cardiac arrest (weak recommendation, low-quality evidence).[9]

Mechanical Cardiopulmonary Resuscitation Devices

When manual CPR is provided by 1 person for more than 2 minutes, the quality deteriorates as the person tires.[23] This led to the 2010 AHA recommendation and best practice of efficiently switching rescuers every 2 minutes.[24] Because prolonged CPR is tiring, the use of a device to deliver compressions is a compelling notion. At the writing of the 2010 recommendations, the evidence regarding the effects of using a mechanical device on outcome was less clear than it is currently. Randomized clinical trials comparing manual and mechanical CPR have shown either no difference in outcome[25] or equivalency[26] and several have shown that the use of the device was associated with harm.[27,28] Additionally, application of the devices may lead to pauses in compressions and in delayed time to defibrillation. Although there is no question that these devices may enable the delivery of high-quality CPR for a sustained period, the bulk of the evidence suggests no significant difference between manual and mechanical chest compressions related to survival from cardiac arrest.

The ILCOR treatment recommendations state

- We suggest against the routine use of automated mechanical chest compression devices to replace manual chest compressions (weak recommendation, moderate-quality evidence).[29]

Clearly, there may be situations in which mechanical devices can provide benefit; however, these situations should be assessed based on all relevant factors in a system.

- We suggest that automated mechanical chest compression devices are a reasonable alternative to high-quality manual chest compressions in situations where sustained high-quality manual chest compressions are impractical or compromise provider safety (weak recommendation, low-quality evidence).[29]

Best Practices

The need for emphasis on high-quality CPR was first described in the 2010 guidelines and treatment recommendations. The importance of focusing on minimizing interruptions, providing effective compressions within the range of recommendations, and avoiding excessive ventilation rates are all discussed previously. Despite the knowledge and recommendations, significant variations persist in outcomes as well as in practices across the country.[30,31] Methods for instituting, monitoring, and improving resuscitation are not in place in many communities, and there remains considerable lack of coordination of care among components of the system.

To provide optimal outcomes for victims of out of hospital SCA, today's best practices must involve the consistent implementation, measurement feedback, and improvement of all aspects of resuscitation care.

MEASUREMENT AND PERFORMANCE IMPROVEMENT

Survival to discharge, in particular survival with good neurologic outcome, is the most significant metric that can be measured in a system, because this provides information about the effectiveness of the system of care in any community. Obtaining outcomes data requires a system of data sharing between the EMS agency and hospitals through a direct exchange of information or through a registry. In the United States, the CARES houses a large and robust collection of data elements pertinent to SCA, including survival measures.[14] Participating in the CARES registry provides multiple actionable metrics that can be invaluable for quality improvement in any system. The ILCOR treatment recommendation for measurement and quality improvement states:

- We suggest the use of performance measurement and quality improvement initiatives in organizations that treat cardiac arrest (weak recommendation, very-low-quality evidence).[32]

It is often stated that only what can be measured can be improved and making the effort to undertake performance measurement and quality-improvement interventions for resuscitation can only help to improve the entire system. Assessing clinical performance and putting into place a system to continuously assess and improve quality can improve adherence to guidelines.[32]

Cardiopulmonary Resuscitation Analytics and Feedback

Poor-quality CPR is a preventable harm, which can be monitored and thus improved through the use of standardized approaches. The major monitor/defibrillator manufacturers offer postevent review software that can capture metrics related to CPR quality, in particular compression and ventilation rates and the occurrence and duration of pauses in CPR. These major components of high-quality CPR contribute to improving blood flow and outcome, and many systems have begun to use these tools in debriefing sessions with the resuscitation teams.

Chest Compression Fraction

CPR analytical software will measure and provide reports documenting the chest compression fraction (CCF), defined as the proportion of time during the resuscitation that compressions are performed. When pauses in CPR during resuscitation are minimized, the CCF is increased. Several studies have shown an association between lower CCFs and worse outcomes of both ROSC and survival,[33] whereas increased CCF is associated with improved survival from out-of-hospital cardiac arrest (OHCA) with shockable rhythms.[7] Postevent review of resuscitation using CPR analytical software to evaluate the quality of CPR is an important aspect of improvement and maintaining high-quality care. The current AHA guidelines recommend a CCF of at least 60%; however, CPR is often performed with CCFs well below that recommendation.[1,3] CCFs of at least 80% are believed achievable and are often cited as an appropriate goal.[34] Some pauses in CPR are unavoidable but should be minimized.

Pauses

CPR analytical software will also allow evaluation of pauses during CPR. Eliminating or significantly minimizing pauses during CPR is a good target for improvement. All pauses should be carefully assessed to ensure they are necessary and should be kept to less than 10 seconds if possible.[34] Numerous strategies to reduce the time without compressions have been devised and should be considered when optimizing CPR.[35]

Postresuscitation Feedback

The AHA does not make any recommendations for focused debriefing after prehospital cardiac arrest resuscitations.[36] A recent study described an increase in CCF and a decrease in duration of chest compression pauses after instituting an OHCA post–code feedback program in Amsterdam.[37] Debriefing sessions and other opportunities for providers to review the resuscitation and receive feedback should be integrated into prehospital systems. In addition to improving patient care, debriefings may offer psychological benefits to responders after critical incidents.[38]

Treatment recommendations from ILCOR include

- We suggest data-driven, performance-focused debriefing of rescuers after OHCA in both adults and children (weak recommendation, very-low-quality evidence).[39]

SUMMARY

A high quality resuscitation requires consistent attention to detail. Short pauses in compressions or unintentional hyperventilation can significantly affect patient outcome. If we are to afford our patients the best possible chance of survival, resuscitation protocols should be consistent across all agencies likely to respond to an out of hospital cardiac arrest; processes should be well established within the entire system of care; and post event review should be used to drive further improvements.

REFERENCES

1. Wik L, Kramer-Johansen J, Myklebust H, et al. Quality of cardiopulmonary resuscitation during out-of-hospital cardiac arrest. JAMA 2005;293:299–304.
2. Brouwer TF, Walker RG, Chapman FW, et al. Association between chest compression interruptions and clinical outcomes of ventricular fibrillation out-of-hospital cardiac arrest. Circulation 2015;132: 1030–7.
3. Kleinman ME, Brennan EE, Goldberger ZD, et al. Part 5: adult basic life support and cardiopulmonary resuscitation quality: 2015 American Heart Association guidelines update for cardiopulmonary resuscitation and emergency cardiovascular care. Circulation 2015;132:S414–35.
4. Berg RA, Hemphill R, Abella BS, et al. Part 5: adult basic life support: 2010 American Heart Association guidelines for cardiopulmonary resuscitation and emergency cardiovascular care. Circulation 2010; 122:S685–705.
5. Kim S, Ahn KO, Jeong S. The effect of team-based cardiopulmonary resuscitation on outcomes in out-of-hospital cardiac arrest patients: a meta-analysis. Am J Emerg Med 2018;36(2):248–52.
6. Olasveengen TM, de Caen AR, Mancini ME, et al. 2017 International consensus on cardiopulmonary resuscitation and emergency cardiovascular care science with treatment recommendations summary. Resuscitation 2017;121:201–14.
7. Christenson J, Andrusiek D, Everson-Stewart S, et al. Chest compression fraction determines survival in patients with out-of-hospital ventricular fibrillation. Circulation 2009;120:1241–7.
8. Idris AH, Guffey D, Pepe PE, et al. Chest compression rates and survival following out-of-hospital cardiac arrest. Crit Care Med 2015;43:840–8.
9. Perkins GD, Travers AH, Berg RA, et al. Part 3: adult basic life support and automated external defibrillation: 2015 International consensus on cardiopulmonary resuscitation and emergency cardiovascular care science with treatment recommendations. Resuscitation 2015;95:e43–69.
10. Fitzgerald KR, Babbs CF, Frissora HA, et al. Cardiac output during cardiopulmonary resuscitation at various compression rates and durations. Am J Physiol 1981;241:H442–8.
11. Zou Y, Shi W, Zhu Y, et al. Rate at 120/min provides qualified chest compression during cardiopulmonary resuscitation. Am J Emerg Med 2015;33:535–8.
12. Nichol G, Leroux B, Wang H, et al. Trial of continuous or interrupted chest compressions during CPR. N Engl J Med 2015;373:2203–14.
13. Bobrow BJ, Clark LL, Ewy GA, et al. Minimally interrupted cardiac resuscitation by emergency medical services for out-of-hospital cardiac arrest. JAMA 2008;299:1158–65.
14. Cardiac arrest registry to enhance survival. 2016 non-traumatic survival rate report. Available at: https://mycares.net. Accessed February 3, 2018.
15. Esibov A, Taylor TG, McInick SB, et al. Controlled pauses ("stutter") CPR did not improve ROSC or 4-hour survival in a porcine model of VF-induced cardiac arrest. Circulation 2015;132:A16996.
16. ECC Committee, Subcommittees and Task Forces of the American Heart Association. 2005 American Heart Association guidelines for cardiopulmonary resuscitation and emergency cardiovascular care. Circulation 2005;112:IV1-203.
17. Vadeboncoeur T, Stolz U, Panchal A, et al. Chest compression depth and survival in out-of-hospital cardiac arrest. Resuscitation 2014;85:182–8.
18. Stiell IG, Brown SP, Nichol G, et al. What is the optimal chest compression depth during out-of-hospital cardiac arrest resuscitation of adult patients? Circulation 2014;130:1962–70.
19. Nikolla DA, Carlson JN. Which compression-to-ventilation ratio yields better cardiac arrest outcomes? Ann Emerg Med 2018;71(4):485–6.
20. O'Neill JF, Deakin CD. Do we hyperventilate cardiac arrest patients? Resuscitation 2007;73:82–5.
21. Aufderheide TP, Lurie KG. Death by hyperventilation: a common and life-threatening problem during cardiopulmonary resuscitation. Crit Care Med 2004; 32:S345–51.
22. Aufderheide TP, Sigurdsson G, Pirrallo RG, et al. Hyperventilation-induced hypotension during cardiopulmonary resuscitation. Circulation 2004;109: 1960–5.
23. Sugarman NT, Herzberg D, Leary M, et al. Rescuer fatigue during actual in-hospital cardiopulmonary resuscitation with audiovisual feedback: a prospective multicenter study. Resuscitation 2009;80(9):981–4.
24. Travers AH, Rea TD, Bobrow BJ, et al. Part 4: CPR overview: 2010 American Heart Association guidelines for cardiopulmonary resuscitation and emergency cardiovascular care. Circulation 2010; 122(18 Suppl 3):S676–84.

25. Rubertsson S, Lindgren E, Smekal D, et al. Per-protocol and pre-defined population analysis of the LINC study. Resuscitation 2015;96:92–9.

26. Wik L, Olsen JA, Persse D, et al. Manual vs. integrated automatic load-distributing band CPR with equal survival after out-of-hospital cardiac arrest. The Randomized CIRC trial. Resuscitation 2014; 85(9):1306.

27. Perkins GD, Handley AJ. Chest compression-only versus standard CPR. Lancet 2011;377(9767):716.

28. Hallstrom A, Rea TD, Sayre MR, et al. Manual chest compression vs use of an automated chest compression device during resuscitation following out-of-hospital cardiac arrest: a randomized trial. JAMA 2006;295(22):2620–8.

29. Soar J, Nolan JP, Böttiger BW, et al. European resuscitation council guidelines for resuscitation 2015: section 3. Adult advanced life support. Resuscitation 2015;95:100–47.

30. Nichol G, Thomas E, Callaway CW, et al. Regional variation in out-of-hospital cardiac arrest incidence and outcome. JAMA 2008;300(12):1423–31.

31. Perkins GD, Cooke MW. Variability in cardiac arrest survival: the NHS ambulance service quality indicators. Emerg Med J 2012;29(1):3–5.

32. Vaillancourt C, Everson-Stewart S, Christenson J, et al. The impact of increased chest compression fraction on return of spontaneous circulation for out-of-hospital cardiac arrest patients not in ventricular fibrillation. Resuscitation 2011;82(12):1501–7.

33. Cheskes S, Schmicker RH, Verbeek PR, et al. The impact of peri-shock pause on survival from out-of hospital shockable cardiac arrest during the resuscitation outcomes consortium PRIMED trial. Resuscitation 2014;85:336–42.

34. Meany PA, Bobrow J, Mancini ME, et al. Cardiopulmonary resuscitation quality: improving cardiac resuscitation outcomes both inside and outside the hospital. A consensus statement from the American Heart Association. Circulation 2013;128:417–35.

35. Cheskes S, Common MR, Byers PA, et al. Compressions during defibrillator charging shortens shock pause duration and improves chest compression fraction during shockable out-of-hospital cardiac arrest. Resuscitation 2014;85:1007–11.

36. Kronick SL, Kurz MC, Lin S, et al. Part 4: systems of care and continuous quality improvement: 2015 American Heart Association guidelines update for cardiopulmonary resuscitation and emergency cardiovascular care. Circulation 2015;132: S397–413.

37. Bleijenberg E, Koster RW, de Vries H, et al. The impact of post-resuscitation feedback for paramedics on the quality of cardiopulmonary resuscitation. Resuscitation 2017;110:1–5.

38. Ireland S, Gilchrist J, Maconochie I. Debriefing after failed paediatric resuscitation: a survey of current UK practice. Emerg Med J 2008;25:328–30.

39. Finn JC, Bhanji F, Lockey A, et al. Part 8: education, implementation, and teams: 2015 International consensus on cardiopulmonary resuscitation and emergency cardiovascular care science with treatment recommendations. Resuscitation 2015;95: e203–24.

Drugs in Out-of-Hospital Cardiac Arrest

Timothy Satty, MD, Christian Martin-Gill, MD, MPH*

KEYWORDS

- Cardiac arrest • Emergency medical services • Medications • Advanced cardiac life support

KEY POINTS

- Limited evidence exists regarding the optimal medical therapy for the management of out-of-hospital cardiac arrest.
- Epinephrine is the only recommended medication for all cardiac arrests.
- Amiodarone or lidocaine is recommended for refractory ventricular fibrillation or ventricular tachycardia.
- Although there is evidence that these medications increase short-term survival, there are few data that they affect long-term outcome measures.
- Other medications should only be considered for use in special situations during out-of-hospital cardiac arrest.

INTRODUCTION

More than 350,000 people suffer out-of-hospital cardiac arrest (OHCA) in the United States each year,[1] and 60% of these patients are treated by emergency medical services (EMS).[2] Despite medical advancements, overall survival to hospital discharge continues to be only 11%.[1] Recognition of cardiac arrest and early application of quality cardiopulmonary resuscitation and defibrillation remain the crucial steps to survival from OHCA. Yet, improvements in medical therapies for cardiac arrest have the potential to save tens of thousands of lives every year.

Management of OHCA has distinct differences compared with in-hospital cardiac arrest, including lengthy response times of trained personnel, limited resources on scene, and multiple challenges to implementation of treatment guidelines.[3] Additionally, logistical considerations for EMS-administered medications include ease of administration, storage space, temperature stability, and cost. For example, medications supplied in pre-filled syringes and administered by bolus are more feasible to administer quickly than medications requiring mixing with a diluent or administered by infusion. Unproven or equivalent medical therapies can become distractors in the out-of-hospital setting, where simplified algorithms emphasizing the most important aspects of resuscitation are more likely to result in a return of spontaneous circulation (ROSC) and good patient outcomes. Current evidence-based guidelines for OHCA remain limited by the low quality of available evidence, and most recommendations are based on metaanalyses and systematic reviews of primarily retrospective studies.[4,5] Newer randomized controlled trials (RCTs) performed outside of the hospital have advanced our knowledge substantially, yet RCTs remain a minority of studies on OHCA owing to multiple logistical barriers and high cost.

In this article, we review the literature and highlight some of the key studies that have evaluated

Disclosure: The authors have nothing to disclose.
Department of Emergency Medicine, University of Pittsburgh School of Medicine, Iroquois Building, Suite 400A, 3600 Forbes Avenue, Pittsburgh, PA 15261, USA
* Corresponding author.
E-mail address: martingillc2@upmc.edu

Cardiol Clin 36 (2018) 357–366
https://doi.org/10.1016/j.ccl.2018.03.003

specific medications for the treatment of OHCA. We also summarize evidence-based guidelines from the American Heart Association (AHA),[4,5] which form the basis for EMS protocols for OHCA management in the United States (**Tables 1** and **2**).

VASOPRESSORS
Epinephrine

Epinephrine is an adrenergic agonist that has been used for resuscitation of cardiac arrest since the earliest standardized guidelines.[6] Early animal studies of epinephrine demonstrated improved rates of ROSC[7,8] and improved cerebral and myocardial blood flow during cardiopulmonary resuscitation.[9] The evidence for patient-centered outcomes has been more limited, with the majority of human data being observational. RCTs comparing epinephrine against placebo have been difficult to perform because its use in cardiac arrest has become the standard of care in many areas.

A large observational study in Japan questioned the value of epinephrine in OHCA.[10] In this study of 400,000 cases of OHCA, epinephrine use increased the chance of prehospital ROSC, but there was a negative association between epinephrine and both 1-month survival and 1-month functional outcomes. This study was followed by the only prehospital RCT comparing epinephrine with placebo, performed in Western Australia, which found that epinephrine was significantly associated with prehospital ROSC.[11] Additionally, twice as many patients in the epinephrine group survived to hospital discharge, but this was not statistically significant, possibly owing to the trial being underpowered for this outcome and raising questions

Table 1
American Heart Association recommendations for medications in cardiac arrest

Category	Medication	Indication	IV/IO Dosing	Recommendation (LOE)
Vasopressor	Epinephrine	Any rhythm	1 mg every 3–5 min	Recommended (class IIb, LOE B)
	Vasopressin	Any rhythm	40 U (replacing first or second dose of epinephrine)	No benefit over epinephrine (class IIb, LOE B)
Antiarrhythmic	Amiodarone	VF/pVT	300 mg (first dose) 150 mg (second dose)	Recommended (class IIb, LOE B)
	Lidocaine	VF/pVT	1.5 mg/kg	Recommended (class IIb, LOE C)
	Magnesium sulfate	Polymorphic VT (torsades de pointes)[a]	1–2 g diluted in 10 mL D5W	Recommended (class IIb, LOE C)
		VF/pVT	Not recommended	Not Recommended (class III: no benefit, LOE B)
	Procainamide	VF/pVT (as second agent)	500 mg, repeated up to 17 mg/kg	Uncertain benefit (not addressed)
	Calcium chloride	Any rhythm	500–1000 mg	Not recommended (class III, LOE B)
	Atropine	Asystole, PEA	1 mg	Not recommended (class IIb, LOE B)
	Sotalol	VF/pVT	1.5 mg/kg	Not addressed
Other	Sodium bicarbonate	Any rhythm	1 mEq/kg	Not recommended (class III, LOE B)
	Naloxone	Any rhythm	2 mg	No Recommendation[b]

Abbreviations: D5W, dextrose 5% in water; LOE, level of evidence; PEA, pulseless electrical activity; pVT, pulseless ventricular tachycardia; VF, ventricular fibrillation; VT, ventricular tachycardia.
[a] Recommended only when polymorphic VT is associated with a long QT interval.
[b] No recommendation for confirmed cardiac arrest.
Data from Link MS, Berkow LC, Kudenchuk PJ, et al. Part 7: Adult advanced cardiovascular life support: 2015 American Heart Association guidelines update for cardiopulmonary resuscitation and emergency cardiovascular care. Circulation 2015;132(18 Suppl 2):S444–64.

Table 2
Recommended medications for special circumstances of cardiac arrest

Indication Associated with Cardiac Arrest	Recommendation	Strength of Recommendation and LOE
Anaphylaxis	Alternate vasoactive drugs (vasopressin, norepinephrine, methoxamine, and metaraminol), and adjuvant use of antihistamines, inhaled beta-adrenergic agents, and IV corticosteroids may be considered	Class IIb, LOE C
Hyperkalemia	Stabilize myocardial cell membrane: Calcium chloride (10%) 5–10 mL (500–1000 mg), or calcium gluconate (10%) 15–30 mL. Shift potassium into cells: Sodium bicarbonate 50 mEq IV over 5 min. Dextrose (50%) 25 g IV and regular insulin 10 U IV over 15–30 min	Class IIb, LOE C
Hypokalemia	Standard resuscitation	Class III, LOE C (for administering potassium)
Hypernatremia	Standard resuscitation	No evidence
Hypermagnesemia	Calcium chloride (10%) 5–10 mL (500–1000 mg), or calcium gluconate (10%) 15–30 mL	Class IIb, LOE C
Hypomagnesemia	Magnesium sulfate 1–2 g IV	Class I, LOE C
Hypercalcemia	Standard resuscitation	No evidence
Hypocalcemia	Standard resuscitation	No evidence
Opioid overdose	Naloxone 2 mg IM/IN may be administered by first aid and non–health care providers; no benefit in confirmed cardiac arrest	Class IIb, LOE C
Other toxic ingestion	Standard resuscitation	No evidence
Hypothermia	Consider administration of a vasopressor during cardiac arrest according to the standard algorithm	Class IIb, LOE C
Polymorphic ventricular tachycardia (torsades de pointes)	Magnesium sulfate 1–2 g IV	Class I, LOE C

Abbreviations: IV, intravenous; LOE, level of evidence.

Data from Lavonas EJ, Drennan IR, Gabrielli A, et al. Part 10: Special circumstances of resuscitation: 2015 American Heart Association guidelines update for cardiopulmonary resuscitation and emergency cardiovascular care. Circulation 2015;132(18 Suppl 2):S501–18; and Vanden Hoek TL, Morrison LJ, Shuster M, et al. Part 12: Cardiac arrest in special situations: 2010 American Heart Association guidelines for cardiopulmonary resuscitation and emergency cardiovascular care. Circulation 2010;122(18 Suppl 3):S829–61.

about benefit in long-term outcomes. Demonstrating the present challenge with studying epinephrine, some EMS systems within this multicenter trial dropped out of participation owing to concerns of withholding a "standard of care" medication. Even in agencies that participated, participation in the study by individual paramedics was voluntary with only 40% of eligible patients recruited to participate.

Three systematic reviews and metaanalyses have aimed to synthesize the data on epinephrine for OHCA. These have focused on only RCTs involving epinephrine in OHCA,[12] or included both observational studies and RCTs.[13,14] These investigations identified that epinephrine seems to have a positive effect on attainment of short-term outcomes such as ROSC but not for long-term survival or neurologic outcomes. Additionally, multiple RCTs comparing standard with high-dose epinephrine did not show significant improvements in survival to discharge.[15–20]

American Heart Association recommendation
Epinephrine remains the principal medication recommended for cardiac arrest for all rhythms, at a dose of 1 mg every 3 to 5 minutes.[4]

Vasopressin

Vasopressin has previously been recommended as an alternative vasopressor to replace the first or second dose of epinephrine in cardiac arrest.[21] It operates on a separate receptor from epinephrine and has better stability in acidic environments.[22] Animal studies have shown improved coronary perfusion pressure, ROSC, and myocardial blood flow compared with epinephrine.[23–25] However, human studies comparing its effectiveness with epinephrine have drawn mixed conclusions. Early studies suggested improvements in ROSC and 24-hour survival in patients receiving vasopressin versus epinephrine alone,[26,27] but no difference in survival to discharge.[27] A 2005 metaanalysis that included 5 RCTs of both in-hospital cardiac arrest and OHCA found no advantage to vasopressin compared with epinephrine in ROSC, survival to discharge, or death at 24 hours.[28] Two additional RCTs of OHCA patients found no significant difference in ROSC, 24-hour survival, or survival to discharge.[29,30] Two subsequent systematic reviews and metaanalyses in 2012 and 2014 also failed to find improvement in rates of sustained ROSC, long-term survival, or survival with favorable neurologic outcomes.[12,31] A metaanalysis by Mentzelopoulos and colleagues[31] did note an increased probability of long-term survival among those patients in asystole, especially when looking at patients with an average time to drug of less than 20 minutes. Overall, data on the use of vasopressin for OHCA suggest no improvement in long-term patient outcomes compared with epinephrine alone. Administering vasopressin as a part of a prehospital protocol adds complexity, cost, and potential distraction from other higher value interventions.

American Heart Association recommendation
Current AHA guidelines no longer include vasopressin as a recommended medication for cardiac arrest.[4]

ANTIARRHYTHMIC AGENTS
Lidocaine

Antiarrhythmic medications are commonly used to promote successful defibrillation of refractory ventricular fibrillation (VF) or pulseless ventricular tachycardia (VT). Despite the widespread use of lidocaine for this indication, there are limited low-quality data addressing its use in the out-of-hospital setting. An observational study published in 1981 compared the survival of prehospital patients who did or did not receive lidocaine for the treatment of refractory VF.[32] This small uncontrolled study (n = 116) found a nonsignificant increase in survival to admission and survival to hospital discharge in patients who received lidocaine. A subsequent 1997 retrospective review of 1212 cardiac arrest patients found that those who received lidocaine had a higher rate of ROSC and were more likely to survive to admission, but there was no significant difference in survival to discharge.[33] Two recent systematic reviews and metaanalyses found that lidocaine was associated with a statistically significant increase in ROSC and survival to admission compared with placebo, but no significant difference in survival to hospital discharge or neurologically intact survival.[34,35]

Amiodarone

Amiodarone has also been widely used as an antiarrhythmic agent in cardiac arrest with limited outcome data supporting its use. An RCT of amiodarone versus placebo for refractory ventricular tachydysrhythmias found that significantly more patients who received amiodarone survived to hospital admission, without a difference in survival to discharge.[36] Similar to lidocaine, 2 systematic reviews and metaanalyses demonstrated an association between amiodarone administration and ROSC or survival to admission compared with placebo, but not to survival to hospital discharge or favorable neurologic outcome.[34,35]

Lidocaine Versus Amiodarone

Several studies have aimed to compare the effectiveness of lidocaine versus amiodarone for refractory ventricular arrhythmias. An RCT comparing amiodarone versus lidocaine found more patients in the amiodarone group survived to admission (22% vs 12%), but no difference in survival to discharge.[37] Shorter time from dispatch to administration of the drug also improved survival to admission, suggesting that some of the benefit of these antiarrhythmics may be diluted by delays in drug administration during OHCA management. The large multi-center Amiodarone, Lidocaine, or Placebo Study (ALPS) confirmed earlier findings of an increased rate of survival to admission with either antiarrhythmic, but there was no increase in survival to hospital discharge or discharge with favorable neurologic outcome with either drug compared with placebo.[38] However, patients with witnessed cardiac arrest were more likely to survive to discharge if they had received either antiarrhythmic medication and patients who had an EMS-witnessed arrest had a higher survival rate with amiodarone versus placebo. No difference was found when comparing amiodarone directly with lidocaine in survival to admission, discharge, or favorable neurologic outcome. A 2016 metaanalysis that included the ALPS study found no difference in survival to admission or discharge when comparing amiodarone with lidocaine.[34] Overall, studies have been consistent in showing that amiodarone and lidocaine improve short-term survival, but have a more limited or no benefit in long-term survival. However, in the largest randomized study performed to date, a long-term survival advantage of antiarrhythmic medications was significant in witnessed prehospital arrest patients.[38]

American Heart Association recommendation

Current AHA guidelines continue to recommend the administration of amiodarone for refractory VF or pulseless VT, and lidocaine may be considered as an alternative to amiodarone for this indication.[4]

Procainamide

Procainamide has also been considered for use in cardiac arrest based on evidence showing its ability to terminate VT in stable patients,[39] but limited data are available regarding its use in OHCA. In a 1995 observational study of in-hospital cardiac arrest and OHCA, a small subset of 20 patients who received procainamide had a significantly increased rate of 1-hour survival and survival to discharge, but the small number of cases makes this estimate uncertain.[40] A 10-year study of 665 patients with OHCA found that when controlling for confounders and other medications administered, patients who received procainamide (n = 176) had no difference in survival to hospital discharge.[41]

American Heart Association recommendation

The use of procainamide for cardiac arrest is not recommended, given the lack of data on its effectiveness.[4]

Magnesium

The use of magnesium as an antiarrhythmic in cardiac arrest has followed case reports of its use after prolonged downtimes with patient survival.[42,43] Magnesium has also been used successfully as a treatment for terminating polymorphic VT with a prolonged QT interval (ie, torsades de pointes).[44,45] A small trial randomized

67 cardiac arrest patients to receive 5 g of magnesium sulfate or placebo as the first medication given upon arrival regardless of rhythm.[46] Four patients from each group survived to be admitted, with no significant differences between groups. Similarly, an in-hospital cardiac arrest study that randomized patients to receive magnesium or placebo failed to find a significant difference in ROSC or 24-hour survival.[47] Another prehospital RCT of patients with refractory VF randomized patients to receive magnesium with the first dose of epinephrine or placebo and found no difference in ROSC, survival to admission, or survival to discharge.[48] The authors performed a metaanalysis, pooling data from prior studies, and had similar conclusions.

American Heart Association recommendation

The routine administration of magnesium in cardiac arrest is not recommended, but it may be used for polymorphic VT with a prolonged QT interval.[4]

Atropine

Atropine has been recommended previously for the management of cardiac arrest associated with asystole or pulseless electrical activity.[49] Atropine is presumed to remove excess vagal tone, which may contribute to cardiac arrest associated with these rhythms,[49] but prospective and randomized controlled trials evaluating atropine use are limited. A small 1981 study randomized patients in asystole or slow idioventricular rhythms to receive atropine or other usual advanced cardiac life support care and found no difference in outcomes compared with usual advanced cardiac life support care alone.[50] A secondary analysis of an RCT evaluating high-dose versus a standard dose of epinephrine found that atropine use was not associated with improved ROSC or survival to discharge.[40] However, there was a correlation with better survival when atropine was given late in the resuscitation. In contrast, a 1998 prospective cohort study of patients with an in-hospital cardiac arrest found a negative association between atropine administration and ROSC when controlling for other patient factors.[51]

The SOS-KANTO study (Survey of Survivors After Out-of-hospital Cardiac Arrest in Kanto Area, Japan) used data from a large observational study of OHCA patients transported to 58 hospitals in Japan and compared patients who received epinephrine alone or epinephrine with atropine.[52] In patients with asystole, the atropine group had significantly increased rates of ROSC and survival to admission but not survival at 30 days or favorable neurologic outcomes. In patients with pulseless electrical activity, there was no survival benefit associated with atropine usage.

American Heart Association recommendation
The routine use of atropine in cardiac arrest is not recommended, regardless of rhythm.[21]

Calcium

The bulk of human data on calcium administration in OHCA comes from limited studies mostly from the 1980s, based on the proposed physiologic mechanism of increasing myocardial contractility. Several small retrospective studies of calcium in patients with pulseless electrical activity or asystole found no significant benefit in ROSC or long-term survival.[53–55] However, a subgroup of patients in pulseless electrical activity with a widened QRS, peaked T waves, or elevated ST segments identified a significant effect of calcium compared with placebo in ROSC, but not in survival to hospital discharge.[55] More recently, a systematic review on calcium administration during cardiac arrest noted small sample sizes across studies, few survivors to discharge, and no strong data to support its use.[56]

Calcium has been suggested in the treatment of cardiac arrest associated with hyperkalemia owing to its ability to stabilize myocardial cell membranes.[57] In a retrospective study of patients with in-hospital cardiac arrest and documented hyperkalemia, bicarbonate and calcium given together was associated with ROSC when the potassium level was less than 9.4 mEq/L.[58] There were not enough patients to review the effect of calcium alone. Calcium has also been considered for the treatment of cardiac arrest secondary to hypermagnesemia, calcium channel blocker overdoses, or beta-blocker overdoses, but there is a lack of substantive data to support any of those indications.[57]

American Heart Association recommendation
The routine administration of calcium for the treatment of cardiac arrest is not recommended.[4] Calcium may be considered for cardiac arrest with suspected hyperkalemia.[57,59]

Beta-Blockers

Beta-blockers may be helpful for terminating recurring VF or VT by blunting sympathetic response.[60] A 2000 prospective study of patients with recurrent VF or VT after myocardial infarction found that patients receiving a beta-blocker or a left stellate ganglion block for sympathetic blockade had significantly less mortality at 1 week,[60] although this study did not assess the ability of beta-blockers to acutely terminate a lethal rhythm. Another study enrolled 42 consecutive patients in VF/VT resistant to a class III antiarrhythmic drug, and found conversion of VF/VT in 79% of patients after the administration of landiolol, with the majority surviving to discharge.[61] Additionally, an RCT in OHCA evaluated sotalol versus lidocaine for VF refractory to 4 or more defibrillations.[62] There was no difference in survival to hospital admission or discharge. A 2012 systematic review identified that the majority of data on the use of beta-blockers in cardiac arrest came from animal data, case reports, or small case series, with the only prospective human data from the previously mentioned trials.[63] The authors concluded that the data points toward a beneficial effect of beta-blockade in patients with cardiac arrest from a shockable rhythm, but more high-quality trials are needed.

American Heart Association recommendation
Current AHA guidelines provide no recommendation regarding use of beta-blockers in cardiac arrest.[4]

OTHER MEDICATIONS
Sodium Bicarbonate

The use of sodium bicarbonate in cardiac arrest was recommended in the first advanced cardiac life support standards in an attempt to reverse the acidemia that develops when perfusion stops.[6] However, evidence on the efficacy of sodium bicarbonate in cardiac arrest has been mixed and generally of low quality. Several observational studies have found no improvement in ROSC or survival to hospital discharge with sodium bicarbonate administration.[40,51,64,65]

A prospective trial randomized OHCA patients to either placebo or a buffer solution (Tribonat) and found no difference in survival to admission or survival to discharge between the 2 groups.[66] Vukmir and colleagues[67] randomized patients who had an OHCA to receive sodium bicarbonate or placebo early in cardiac arrest and found no difference in survival to the ED. The authors did find improvement with bicarbonate in prolonged prehospital cardiac arrest, noting that survival to the ED doubled in patients with more than 15 minutes of downtime. They did not study the effect on long-term survival. A recent review article of human and animal studies found that many studies show little or no benefit and possibly some harm from giving sodium bicarbonate in cardiac arrest.[68]

American Heart Association recommendation
The routine use of sodium bicarbonate in cardiac arrest is not recommended.[4] However, sodium bicarbonate may be beneficial and is recommended

in special situations, such as hyperkalemia, tricyclic antidepressant overdose, or other toxic ingestions.[57]

Naloxone

The opioid epidemic in the United States has resulted in increases in deaths over the past decade.[69] Naloxone works as a potent opioid receptor antagonist and can rapidly reverse respiratory depression, which may precipitate respiratory and cardiac arrest. However, the value of using naloxone once the patient is in cardiac arrest is unclear. Animal studies and case reports on the use of naloxone during cardiac arrest have provided mixed findings, with some suggestion that it may have antiarrhythmic and positive inotropic effects.[70,71] Saybolt and colleagues[71] performed the only known study of naloxone in OHCA. In this retrospective study of 36 patients in cardiac arrest who received naloxone, 42% had improvement in rhythm immediately after administration. However, this study did not compare outcomes in patients managed with and without naloxone administration.

American Heart Association recommendation
The routine use of naloxone by advanced providers in the management of confirmed cardiac arrest is not recommended. However, because first aid and other non–health care providers are not expected to determine if an unresponsive patient is pulseless, empiric administration of naloxone by these providers is reasonable as part of standard resuscitation.[4]

SUMMARY

Challenges to managing OHCA include delays in arrival of trained responders, lack of bystander ability to administer cardiopulmonary resuscitation, and delays in establishment of intravenous access and medication administration, all of which may hinder the potential benefits of medical therapies. For medications to be a beneficial part of out-of-hospital resuscitation, they must have a proven benefit, or they risk acting only as a distraction from proven interventions. Most medications studied for use in OHCA have not been found to have a significant effect on long-term survival. Outside of special situations, only epinephrine is recommended for all cardiac arrest rhythms. Amiodarone or lidocaine are recommended for shock refractory VF or pulseless VT. The routine use of vasopressin, procainamide, magnesium, atropine, calcium, beta-blockers, sodium bicarbonate, or naloxone is not advised based on the available evidence.

REFERENCES

1. Benjamin EJ, Blaha MJ, Chiuve SE, et al. Heart disease and stroke statistics-2017 update: a report from the American Heart Association. Circulation 2017;135(10):e146–603.
2. Go AS, Mozaffarian D, Roger VL, et al. Heart disease and stroke statistics–2013 update: a report from the American Heart Association. Circulation 2013;127(1):e6–245.
3. Bigham BL, Koprowicz K, Aufderheide TP, et al. Delayed prehospital implementation of the 2005 American Heart Association guidelines for cardiopulmonary resuscitation and emergency cardiac care. Prehosp Emerg Care 2010;14(3):355–60.
4. Link MS, Berkow LC, Kudenchuk PJ, et al. Part 7: adult advanced cardiovascular life support: 2015 American Heart Association Guidelines update for cardiopulmonary resuscitation and emergency cardiovascular care. Circulation 2015;132(18 Suppl 2): S444–64.
5. Lavonas EJ, Drennan IR, Gabrielli A, et al. Part 10: special circumstances of resuscitation: 2015 American Heart Association guidelines update for cardiopulmonary resuscitation and emergency cardiovascular care. Circulation 2015;132(18 Suppl 2): S501–18.
6. Standards for Cardiopulmonary Resuscitation (CPR) and Emergency Cardiac Care (ECC). JAMA 1974; 227(7):833–68.
7. Redding JS, Pearson JW. Resuscitation from ventricular fibrillation. Drug therapy. JAMA 1968;203(4): 255–60.
8. Redding JS, Pearson JW. Resuscitation from asphyxia. JAMA 1962;182:283–6.
9. Michael JR, Guerci AD, Koehler RC, et al. Mechanisms by which epinephrine augments cerebral and myocardial perfusion during cardiopulmonary resuscitation in dogs. Circulation 1984;69(4): 822–35.
10. Hagihara A, Hasegawa M, Abe T, et al. Prehospital epinephrine use and survival among patients with out-of-hospital cardiac arrest. JAMA 2012;307(11): 1161–8.
11. Jacobs IG, Finn JC, Jelinek GA, et al. Effect of adrenaline on survival in out-of-hospital cardiac arrest: a randomised double-blind placebo-controlled trial. Resuscitation 2011;82(9):1138–43.
12. Lin S, Callaway CW, Shah PS, et al. Adrenaline for out-of-hospital cardiac arrest resuscitation: a systematic review and meta-analysis of randomized controlled trials. Resuscitation 2014;85(6):732–40.
13. Atiksawedparit P, Rattanasiri S, McEvoy M, et al. Effects of prehospital adrenaline administration on out-of-hospital cardiac arrest outcomes: a systematic review and meta-analysis. Crit Care 2014; 18(4):463.

14. Loomba RS, Nijhawan K, Aggarwal S, et al. Increased return of spontaneous circulation at the expense of neurologic outcomes: is prehospital epinephrine for out-of-hospital cardiac arrest really worth it? J Crit Care 2015;30(6):1376–81.

15. Callaham M, Madsen CD, Barton CW, et al. A randomized clinical trial of high-dose epinephrine and norepinephrine vs standard-dose epinephrine in prehospital cardiac arrest. JAMA 1992;268(19):2667–72.

16. Choux C, Gueugniaud PY, Barbieux A, et al. Standard doses versus repeated high doses of epinephrine in cardiac arrest outside the hospital. Resuscitation 1995;29(1):3–9.

17. Gueugniaud PY, Mols P, Goldstein P, et al. A comparison of repeated high doses and repeated standard doses of epinephrine for cardiac arrest outside the hospital. European Epinephrine Study Group. N Engl J Med 1998;339(22):1595–601.

18. Brown CG, Martin DR, Pepe PE, et al. A comparison of standard-dose and high-dose epinephrine in cardiac arrest outside the hospital. The multicenter high-dose epinephrine study group. N Engl J Med 1992;327(15):1051–5.

19. Sherman BW, Munger MA, Foulke GE, et al. High-dose versus standard-dose epinephrine treatment of cardiac arrest after failure of standard therapy. Pharmacotherapy 1997;17(2):242–7.

20. Stiell IG, Hebert PC, Weitzman BN, et al. High-dose epinephrine in adult cardiac arrest. N Engl J Med 1992;327(15):1045–50.

21. Neumar RW, Otto CW, Link MS, et al. Part 8: adult advanced cardiovascular life support: 2010 American Heart Association guidelines for cardiopulmonary resuscitation and emergency cardiovascular care. Circulation 2010;122(18 Suppl 3):S729–67.

22. Fox AW, May RE, Mitch WE. Comparison of peptide and nonpeptide receptor-mediated responses in rat tail artery. J Cardiovasc Pharmacol 1992;20(2):282–9.

23. Wenzel V, Lindner KH, Krismer AC, et al. Repeated administration of vasopressin but not epinephrine maintains coronary perfusion pressure after early and late administration during prolonged cardiopulmonary resuscitation in pigs. Circulation 1999;99(10):1379–84.

24. Wenzel V, Lindner KH, Prengel AW, et al. Vasopressin improves vital organ blood flow after prolonged cardiac arrest with postcountershock pulseless electrical activity in pigs. Crit Care Med 1999;27(3):486–92.

25. Wenzel V, Lindner KH, Krismer AC, et al. Survival with full neurologic recovery and no cerebral pathology after prolonged cardiopulmonary resuscitation with vasopressin in pigs. J Am Coll Cardiol 2000;35(2):527–33.

26. Guyette FX, Guimond GE, Hostler D, et al. Vasopressin administered with epinephrine is associated with a return of a pulse in out-of-hospital cardiac arrest. Resuscitation 2004;63(3):277–82.

27. Mally S, Jelatancev A, Grmec S. Effects of epinephrine and vasopressin on end-tidal carbon dioxide tension and mean arterial blood pressure in out-of-hospital cardiopulmonary resuscitation: an observational study. Crit Care 2007;11(2):R39.

28. Aung K, Htay T. Vasopressin for cardiac arrest: a systematic review and meta-analysis. Arch Intern Med 2005;165(1):17–24.

29. Callaway CW, Hostler D, Doshi AA, et al. Usefulness of vasopressin administered with epinephrine during out-of-hospital cardiac arrest. Am J Cardiol 2006;98(10):1316–21.

30. Mukoyama T, Kinoshita K, Nagao K, et al. Reduced effectiveness of vasopressin in repeated doses for patients undergoing prolonged cardiopulmonary resuscitation. Resuscitation 2009;80(7):755–61.

31. Mentzelopoulos SD, Zakynthinos SG, Siempos I, et al. Vasopressin for cardiac arrest: meta-analysis of randomized controlled trials. Resuscitation 2012;83(1):32–9.

32. Harrison EE. Lidocaine in prehospital countershock refractory ventricular fibrillation. Ann Emerg Med 1981;10(8):420–3.

33. Herlitz J, Ekstrom L, Wennerblom B, et al. Lidocaine in out-of-hospital ventricular fibrillation. Does it improve survival? Resuscitation 1997;33(3):199–205.

34. Sanfilippo F, Corredor C, Santonocito C, et al. Amiodarone or lidocaine for cardiac arrest: a systematic review and meta-analysis. Resuscitation 2016;107:31–7.

35. McLeod SL, Brignardello-Petersen R, Worster A, et al. Comparative effectiveness of antiarrhythmics for out-of-hospital cardiac arrest: a systematic review and network meta-analysis. Resuscitation 2017;121:90–7.

36. Kudenchuk PJ, Cobb LA, Copass MK, et al. Amiodarone for resuscitation after out-of-hospital cardiac arrest due to ventricular fibrillation. N Engl J Med 1999;341(12):871–8.

37. Dorian P, Cass D, Schwartz B, et al. Amiodarone as compared with lidocaine for shock-resistant ventricular fibrillation. N Engl J Med 2002;346(12):884–90.

38. Kudenchuk PJ, Daya M, Dorian P. Resuscitation outcomes consortium I. Amiodarone, lidocaine, or placebo in out-of-hospital cardiac arrest. N Engl J Med 2016;375(8):802–3.

39. Gorgels AP, van den Dool A, Hofs A, et al. Comparison of procainamide and lidocaine in terminating sustained monomorphic ventricular tachycardia. Am J Cardiol 1996;78(1):43–6.

40. Stiell IG, Wells GA, Hebert PC, et al. Association of drug therapy with survival in cardiac arrest: limited role of advanced cardiac life support drugs. Acad Emerg Med 1995;2(4):264–73.

41. Markel DT, Gold LS, Allen J, et al. Procainamide and survival in ventricular fibrillation out-of-hospital cardiac arrest. Acad Emerg Med 2010;17(6):617–23.

42. Craddock L, Miller B, Clifton G, et al. Resuscitation from prolonged cardiac arrest with high-dose intravenous magnesium sulfate. J Emerg Med 1991; 9(6):469–76.

43. Tobey RC, Birnbaum GA, Allegra JR, et al. Successful resuscitation and neurologic recovery from refractory ventricular fibrillation after magnesium sulfate administration. Ann Emerg Med 1992; 21(1):92–6.

44. Tzivoni D, Banai S, Schuger C, et al. Treatment of torsade de pointes with magnesium sulfate. Circulation 1988;77(2):392–7.

45. Manz M, Jung W, Luderitz B. Effect of magnesium on sustained ventricular tachycardia. Herz 1997; 22(Suppl 1):51–5 [in German].

46. Fatovich DM, Prentice DA, Dobb GJ. Magnesium in cardiac arrest (the magic trial). Resuscitation 1997; 35(3):237–41.

47. Thel MC, Armstrong AL, McNulty SE, et al. Randomised trial of magnesium in in-hospital cardiac arrest. Duke internal medicine housestaff. Lancet 1997;350(9087):1272–6.

48. Allegra J, Lavery R, Cody R, et al. Magnesium sulfate in the treatment of refractory ventricular fibrillation in the prehospital setting. Resuscitation 2001; 49(3):245–9.

49. ECC Committee, Subcommittees and Task Forces of the American Heart Association. 2005 American Heart Association guidelines for cardiopulmonary resuscitation and emergency cardiovascular care. Circulation 2005;112(24 Suppl):IV1–203.

50. Coon GA, Clinton JE, Ruiz E. Use of atropine for brady-asystolic prehospital cardiac arrest. Ann Emerg Med 1981;10(9):462–7.

51. van Walraven C, Stiell IG, Wells GA, et al. Do advanced cardiac life support drugs increase resuscitation rates from in-hospital cardiac arrest? The OTAC study group. Ann Emerg Med 1998;32(5): 544–53.

52. Survey of Survivors After Out-of-hospital Cardiac Arrest in Kanto Area, Japan (SOS-KANTO) Study Group. Atropine sulfate for patients with out-of-hospital cardiac arrest due to asystole and pulseless electrical activity. Circ J 2011;75(3):580–8.

53. Stueven H, Thompson BM, Aprahamian C, et al. Use of calcium in prehospital cardiac arrest. Ann Emerg Med 1983;12(3):136–9.

54. Stueven HA, Thompson B, Aprahamian C, et al. Lack of effectiveness of calcium chloride in refractory asystole. Ann Emerg Med 1985;14(7):630–2.

55. Stueven HA, Thompson B, Aprahamian C, et al. The effectiveness of calcium chloride in refractory electromechanical dissociation. Ann Emerg Med 1985; 14(7):626–9.

56. Kette F, Ghuman J, Parr M. Calcium administration during cardiac arrest: a systematic review. Eur J Emerg Med 2013;20(2):72–8.

57. Vanden Hoek TL, Morrison LJ, Shuster M, et al. Part 12: cardiac arrest in special situations: 2010 American Heart Association guidelines for cardiopulmonary resuscitation and emergency cardiovascular care. Circulation 2010;122(18 Suppl 3):S829–61.

58. Wang CH, Huang CH, Chang WT, et al. The effects of calcium and sodium bicarbonate on severe hyperkalaemia during cardiopulmonary resuscitation: a retrospective cohort study of adult in-hospital cardiac arrest. Resuscitation 2016;98:105–11.

59. Soar J, Perkins GD, Abbas G, et al. European Resuscitation Council Guidelines for Resuscitation 2010 Section 8. Cardiac arrest in special circumstances: electrolyte abnormalities, poisoning, drowning, accidental hypothermia, hyperthermia, asthma, anaphylaxis, cardiac surgery, trauma, pregnancy, electrocution. Resuscitation 2010;81(10): 1400–33.

60. Nademanee K, Taylor R, Bailey WE, et al. Treating electrical storm : sympathetic blockade versus advanced cardiac life support-guided therapy. Circulation 2000;102(7):742–7.

61. Miwa Y, Ikeda T, Mera H, et al. Effects of landiolol, an ultra-short-acting beta1-selective blocker, on electrical storm refractory to class III antiarrhythmic drugs. Circ J 2010;74(5):856–63.

62. Kovoor P, Love A, Hall J, et al. Randomized double-blind trial of sotalol versus lignocaine in out-of-hospital refractory cardiac arrest due to ventricular tachyarrhythmia. Intern Med J 2005; 35(9):518–25.

63. de Oliveira FC, Feitosa-Filho GS, Ritt LE. Use of beta-blockers for the treatment of cardiac arrest due to ventricular fibrillation/pulseless ventricular tachycardia: a systematic review. Resuscitation 2012;83(6):674–83.

64. Delooz HH, Lewi PJ. Are inter-center differences in EMS-management and sodium-bicarbonate administration important for the outcome of CPR? The Cerebral Resuscitation Study Group. Resuscitation 1989;17(Suppl):S161–72 [discussion: S199–206].

65. Weng YM, Wu SH, Li WC, et al. The effects of sodium bicarbonate during prolonged cardiopulmonary resuscitation. Am J Emerg Med 2013;31(3): 562–5.

66. Dybvik T, Strand T, Steen PA. Buffer therapy during out-of-hospital cardiopulmonary resuscitation. Resuscitation 1995;29(2):89–95.

67. Vukmir RB, Katz L, Sodium Bicarbonate Study Group. Sodium bicarbonate improves outcome in prolonged prehospital cardiac arrest. Am J Emerg Med 2006;24(2):156–61.

68. Velissaris D, Karamouzos V, Pierrakos C, et al. Use of sodium bicarbonate in cardiac arrest: current guidelines and literature review. J Clin Med Res 2016;8(4):277–83.

69. Rudd RA, Aleshire N, Zibbell JE, et al. Increases in drug and opioid overdose deaths–United States, 2000-2014. MMWR Morb Mortal Wkly Rep 2016; 64(50–51):1378–82.

70. Martins HS, Silva RV, Bugano D, et al. Should naloxone be prescribed in the ED management of patients with cardiac arrest? A case report and review of literature. Am J Emerg Med 2008;26(1): 113.e5-8.

71. Saybolt MD, Alter SM, Dos Santos F, et al. Naloxone in cardiac arrest with suspected opioid overdoses. Resuscitation 2010;81(1):42–6.

Controversial Issues
Pro Mechanical Cardiopulmonary Resuscitation

Kylie Dyson, PhD[a,b,*], Dion Stub, MBBS, PhD[b,c,d,e],
Stephen Bernard, MBBS, MD[b,e], Karen Smith, PhD[a,b,f]

KEYWORDS

- Cardiopulmonary resuscitation • Out-of-hospital cardiac arrest • Emergency medical services
- Mechanical chest compressions • Equipment

KEY POINTS

- Mechanical chest compressions prevent paramedics from providing unsafe cardiopulmonary resuscitation (CPR) during transport.
- Mechanical chest compressions enable high-quality CPR in difficult situations, for example, extrication and transport.
- Mechanical chest compressions can provide a bridge to treatment of reversible causes of cardiac arrest.

INTRODUCTION

Cardiopulmonary resuscitation (CPR) is unequivocally associated with improved outcomes for patients in out-of-hospital cardiac arrest (OHCA).[1] High-quality CPR, in particular chest compressions, is a key aspect of out-of-hospital cardiac arrest resuscitation.[2] Chest compressions that are performed at the recommended rate and depth with full release and minimal interruptions are associated with improved rates of OHCA survival.[2] Maintaining high-quality chest compressions, throughout prolonged resuscitation in varying conditions of the prehospital environment, is difficult. Therefore, paramedics do not consistently achieve this standard.[3] Therefore, several mechanical devices have been developed as a means of providing consistent, high-quality chest compressions.[4]

Mechanical chest compression devices have been available for decades but have only recently gained widespread adoption internationally by emergency medical services (EMS).[5] These devices provide a theoretic advantage over conventional chest compressions in that they can potentially administer consistent chest compressions according to guideline recommendations. In addition to providing a consistent depth, rate, and release, mechanical chest compression devices remove some human factors, such as fatigue or distraction by other resuscitation interventions and responders (**Figs. 1** and **2**).

Disclosure: The authors have nothing to disclose.
[a] Centre for Research and Evaluation, Ambulance Victoria, 375 Manningham Road, Doncaster, VIC 3108, Australia; [b] Department of Epidemiology and Preventive Medicine, Monash University, 99 Commercial Road, Melbourne, VIC 3004, Australia; [c] Cardiology Department, Alfred Hospital, 55 Commercial Road, Melbourne, VIC 3004, Australia; [d] Cardiology Department, Western Health, Gordon Street, Footscray, VIC 3011, Australia; [e] Medical Directorate, Ambulance Victoria, 375 Manningham Road, Doncaster, VIC 3108, Australia; [f] Department of Community Emergency Health and Paramedic Practice, Monash University, McMahons Road, Frankston, VIC 3199, Australia
* Corresponding author. Centre for Research and Evaluation, Ambulance Victoria, 375 Manningham Road, Doncaster, VIC 3108, Australia.
E-mail address: Kylie.Dyson@ambulance.vic.gov.au

Cardiol Clin 36 (2018) 367–374
https://doi.org/10.1016/j.ccl.2018.03.004

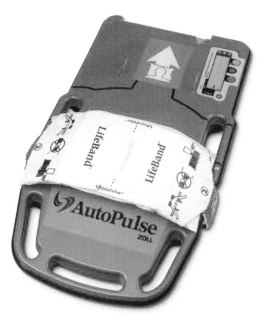

Fig. 1. The AutoPulse Resuscitation System manufactured by Zoll Medical Corporation. This device compresses the chest by tightening a band around the thorax, increasing intrathoracic pressure, and expelling blood from the chest cavity. (*Courtesy of* ZOLL Medical Corporation, Plymouth Meeting, PA.)

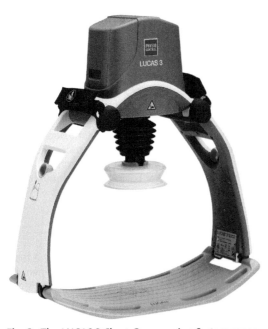

Fig. 2. The LUCAS 3 Chest Compression System manufactured by Physio-Control, Inc. This device uses a piston to compress in a manner similar to that of a human rescuer over the center of the chest to a recommended, preset depth. (*Courtesy of* Physio-Control, Inc, Redmond, WA; with permission.)

There are typically 2 types of mechanical chest compression devices: piston devices and load-distributing band devices. Piston devices consist of a plunger positioned over the sternum which compresses at a set rate. Some piston devices also have a suction cup that is designed to actively decompress the chest after compression. Load-distributing band devices have a circumferential chest compression band which constricts the chest against a backboard. Some chest compression devices, also have radiolucent back plates to facilitate concurrent percutaneous coronary intervention (PCI).

The use of mechanical chest compression devices has been demonstrated as feasible in the prehospital setting; however, as with all medical technology, their application depends on the skill and experience of the provider.[6–8] There is evidence from several studies suggesting that some aspects of chest compression quality can be improved with the implementation of mechanical chest compression devices, particularly chest compression rate and depth.[9,10] However, other studies suggest that mechanical chest compression devices can result in extended pauses in compressions[11–13] and delays to defibrillation.[8,14,15] In particular, CPR fraction and time to defibrillation can be negatively impacted by the time it takes to apply the devices. The significance of this effect often depends on the quality of the manual chest compressions in the comparison group and how early the device is applied during the resuscitation.[13,14]

Animal studies comparing mechanical and manual chest compressions have demonstrated improved cerebral and coronary perfusion.[16–18] Human studies have demonstrated improvements in end-tidal carbon dioxide and regional cerebral oxygenation during mechanical chest compressions.[19–21] In the clinical trial domain, the evidence is more circumspect regarding the routine use of chest compression devices. There have been 4 systematic reviews comparing manual and mechanical chest compressions, using varying inclusion criteria. They concluded that there is no significant difference in survival or neurologic outcome.[22–26] The 5 existing randomized controlled trials (RCTs) comparing manual chest compressions with mechanical devices have found similar survival in both groups.[15,27–30] However, 2 of these RCTs demonstrated a negative association between mechanical chest compressions and good neurologic outcomes[15,28]; one trial was terminated early because of evidence of harm.[15] Possible explanations for these unexpected results include the Hawthorne effect, enrollment bias, study site differences, and the method and timing of applying the device.[14,15,26]

The American Heart Association (AHA) recommends that manual chest compressions remain the standard of care; however, mechanical chest compression devices may be considered in specific settings and circumstances where the delivery of high-quality manual compressions may be challenging or dangerous for the provider.[4] There are many specific settings and circumstances where mechanical chest compression devices provide a useful adjunct to high-quality manual chest compressions.

The AHA suggests[4] that the use of mechanical chest compression devices may be considered in circumstances, such as the following:

- Limited rescuers available
- Prolonged CPR
- During hypothermic cardiac arrest
- In a moving ambulance
- In the angiography suite
- During preparation for extracorporeal CPR

The caveat to this recommendation is that paramedics strictly limit interruptions in CPR during deployment and removal of the devices.[4] In order to achieve this, regular practice would be required given the relatively low exposure to cardiac arrests that paramedics are likely to have[31] and in particular arrests warranting use of mechanical CPR. It is important to emphasize that mechanical chest compression devices in themselves do not resolve the problems associated with poor CPR; paramedics still need to understand the priorities of cardiac arrest resuscitation, including minimizing interruptions during device application.

EXTRICATION, TRANSPORTATION, AND PARAMEDIC SAFETY

One of the most important uses of mechanical chest compression devices is to protect paramedic safety. EMS agencies have a responsibility to protect the welfare of their staff. The extrication and transport of patients in cardiac arrest risks the safety of paramedics and has been shown to undermine the quality of the CPR.[32–34] Many EMS agencies require routine transport of patients in cardiac arrest regardless of whether return of spontaneous circulation (ROSC) is obtained at the scene.[22] The AHA's guidelines for out-of-hospital termination of resuscitation are designed to substantially reduce the rate of emergency EMS transports without appreciably worsening the rate of cardiac arrest survival; however, they still result in a high proportion of patients being transported to the hospital, with ongoing resuscitation.[35–38]

Mechanical chest compression devices reduce the need for paramedics to be unrestrained in the ambulance cabin during transport. A systematic review[39] found that lights and sirens while driving increases the risk of an ambulance crash and paramedics standing increases the risk of injury and death. Mechanical chest compression devices may reduce the risk posed to paramedics during high-speed transports. Crash tests of one mechanical chest compression device demonstrated that it stayed attached during 30 km/h crashes.[7] In addition, these devices eliminate the need to rotate the paramedic performing chest compressions, which may be difficult because of the confined space and limited personnel in the vehicle. This point equally applies to safely and effectively treating patients who rearrest during transport to the hospital.

EMS providers have reported that it is difficult to maintain balance and concurrently deliver CPR while traveling in an ambulance and during extrication.[40] Studies have demonstrated that the quality of manual chest compressions during transport is poor and the delivery of high-quality chest compressions in a moving ambulance is challenging.[32–34] When manual and mechanical chest compressions have been compared during transport in an ambulance, studies have shown that CPR quality is significantly better with mechanical chest compressions, particularly during braking and change maneuvers.[32,41–44]

CPR during helicopter or fixed-wing transportation is particularly challenging. Many EMS agencies that service rural areas use helicopter or fixed-wing transportation to ensure that patients with ST elevation myocardial infarction or ROSC receive timely transport to PCI hospitals. Should these patients or others have a cardiac arrest or rearrest during transport, chest compressions are required. One study found that performing manual chest compressions during helicopter transport was barely possible and only of poor quality but that mechanical chest compression devices are a good alternative in terms of compression rate, depth, and fraction.[45] Mechanical chest compressions during helicopter flights are feasible and can enable rapid transfer of patients so that they can receive further treatment.[46]

LIMITED RESOURCES AND FATIGUE

Two advantages of the mechanical chest compression devices are that they do not fatigue and they enable paramedics to focus on other aspects of patient care. These advantages may be particularly important in settings where limited paramedics are available, such as in rural areas. Studies have demonstrated that fatigue can affect the quality of CPR after only 1 minute of chest compressions and health care professionals are unable to accurately identify the point at which they become fatigued.[47,48] Therefore, in situations whereby few paramedics are available, they may perform manual chest compressions past the point of fatigue, resulting in poor-quality CPR. In addition, mechanical chest compression devices free up paramedics to perform other interventions, such as advanced airway and intravenous insertion, or drug administration.

BRIDGE TO TREATMENT OF REVERSIBLE CAUSES

Given that mechanical chest compressions enable safe and effective CPR during transport, they provide patients with the opportunity to be transported to hospital for treatment of reversible causes of OHCA. Examples of patients with may benefit from hospital interventions include patients with cardiac arrest due to hypothermia or patients in refractory ventricular fibrillation (VF) that may benefit from PCI, or emergent pulmonary embolectomy. Although there is uncertainty around specifically which OHCA patients will benefit from definitive in-hospital treatment, several case series and case reports provide examples in which such treatment has been effective.

PERCUTANEOUS CORONARY INTERVENTION

The fifth link in the chain of cardiac arrest survival is postresuscitation care, including PCI in patients suspected of experiencing myocardial infarction.[49] The AHA recommends emergency coronary angiography for all patients after experiencing cardiac arrest with ST elevation and for unstable patients for whom a cardiovascular lesion is suspected.[50] However, there may be some patients who would benefit from PCI before the postresuscitation stage, while they are still in cardiac arrest. VF is associated with myocardial infarction caused by acute coronary occlusion.[51] Successful PCI performed immediately after ROSC is associated with improved survival for patients with OHCA[52–56]; therefore, PCI may benefit patients still in cardiac arrest, particularly those in VF.[56,57] Mechanical chest compression devices can provide a bridge between the prehospital and hospital environments to enable patients with OHCA to access PCI. In addition, some mechanical chest compression devices have a radiolucent backboard and PCI with ongoing mechanical CPR is feasible.[58–60] These patients need a safe and effective means of connecting to definitive hospital care.

One case study of an OHCA in Italy demonstrates that mechanical chest compression devices can be used to facilitate safe and effective chest compressions during the transfer of a patient by helicopter to a PCI hospital for immediate catheterization.[61] This patient achieved ROSC during PCI, after nearly 2 hours in cardiac arrest. The patient was treated with therapeutic hypothermia in the intensive care unit and survived without any neurologic deficit. Given that manual chest compressions were not possible in the helicopter and road transport would have led to significant delays, this case study reveals how mechanical chest compression devices open up treatment options and survival outcomes not previously thought possible.

EXTRACORPOREAL MEMBRANE OXYGENATION

Few EMS agencies are set up to provide prehospital extracorporeal membrane oxygenation (ECMO); however, many hospitals have specialist teams able to apply ECMO in emergency situations.[62] Transport of patients with OHCA, with a mechanical chest compression device, to a hospital with an ECMO team opens patients up to a broader range of interventions and buys time for such treatments.

One example of mechanical chest compressions being used as a means of safely transporting patients in refractory VF for ECMO, PCI and further treatment is the CHEER (mechanical CPR, Hypothermia, ECMO and Early Reperfusion) trial[63] conducted in the Australian state of Victoria. Paramedics in Victoria rarely transport patients requiring ongoing CPR due to perceived futility and safety concerns.[64] In this study, 11 select OHCAs with refractory VF that had not achieved ROSC after 30 minutes of resuscitation (including advanced life support) received a treatment bundle including mechanical chest compressions, prehospital intra-arrest therapeutic hypothermia, ECMO and rapid coronary angiography. Of the 11 patients with OHCA who participated in this study, 5 (45%) were discharged alive with a good neurologic status. Although this was a small feasibility study, the CHEER trial highlights that, as part of a treatment bundle, mechanical chest compressions provide an opportunity to save the lives of patients who would previously have been declared deceased at scene by paramedics.

A recent trial in Minnesota in 62 patients with refractory VF OHCA, using a similar treatment pathway, reported 42% survival with good neurologic outcomes.[65] The growing adoption of mechanical chest compression devices increases the possibilities for OHCA management and opens up treatment options frequently not available because prolonged resuscitation is often considered futile. The median time from collapse to ECMO in the CHEER[63] and Minnesota[65] studies was 56 and 64 minutes, respectively, revealing that patients can survive a resuscitation that takes much longer than health care professionals are willing or able to perform manual chest compressions. Similar case series in European and North American settings have also demonstrated that using mechanical chest compressions to transition patients with OHCA to ECMO for further in-hospital treatment is feasible and can result in favorable outcomes.[66,67]

TREATMENT OF OTHER REVERSIBLE CAUSES

In addition to patients with OHCA due to coronary occlusion, patients with OHCA due to other potentially reversible causes, such as hypothermia, intoxication, and pulmonary embolism, may benefit from transport to hospital with mechanical chest compressions. For example, patients with OHCA caused by hypothermia may benefit from ECMO and therapeutic hypothermia or rewarming in the intensive care unit,[68–70] a level of intervention that cannot be provided in the field.

One case study of 3 patients with OHCA due to submersion and hypothermia in Sweden after their car crashed into an icy canal illustrates how a mechanical chest compression device may be used to treat OHCA requiring prolonged resuscitation.[70] One patient, who was submersed for approximately 21 minutes and presenting in asystole, was transported to the hospital with ongoing mechanical chest compressions. On arrival at the hospital, the patient was still in asystole and had a temperature of 28°C. ROSC was obtained 47 minutes after the accident; the patient was rewarmed to 33°C, which was maintained for 24 hours in the intensive care unit. The patient was discharged from the hospital with a full recovery. The two other patients who received manual chest compressions to the hospital did not survive.

Another case study of a patient with OHCA due to pulmonary embolism in France shows how a mechanical chest compression device may be used for prolonged resuscitation to enable the treatment of reversible causes to take effect.[71] A patient experiencing sudden chest pain and severe dyspnea had an OHCA witnessed by EMS. Based on suspicion of a pulmonary embolism, the patient was treated with prehospital thrombolysis and mechanical chest compressions; ROSC was obtained 75 minutes after the patient collapsed. In the hospital bilateral pulmonary embolism was confirmed, and the patient was subsequently discharged with a good neurologic condition.

Although the aforementioned examples are only small case series and single case studies, they demonstrate the potential of mechanical chest compression devices to enable prolonged resuscitation and definitive in-hospital treatment of reversible causes with good neurologic outcomes for select patients with specific presentations.

SUMMARY

Regardless of the method used, the objective of EMS agencies is to provide high-quality CPR and maximize the likelihood of a good patient outcome. Therefore, in circumstances whereby high-quality manual chest compressions are difficult or unsafe, paramedics should consider using a mechanical device. Mechanical chest compression devices enable prolonged resuscitation and definitive in-hospital treatment of reversible causes of OHCA for select patients with specific presentations. It is vital that paramedics receive adequate training in the application and removal of chest compression devices and that they are only used in circumstances whereby high-quality manual chest compressions are challenging. By combining high-quality manual chest compressions and judicious application of mechanical chest compressions, EMS agencies can optimize paramedic safety and patient outcomes.

REFERENCES

1. Sasson C, Rogers MAM, Dahl J, et al. Predictors of survival from out-of-hospital cardiac arrest: a systematic review and meta-analysis. Circ Cardiovasc Qual Outcomes 2010;3(1):63–81.
2. Travers AH, Perkins GD, Berg RA, et al. Part 3: adult basic life support and automated external defibrillation: 2015 international consensus on cardiopulmonary resuscitation and emergency cardiovascular care science with treatment recommendations. Circulation 2015;132(16 Suppl 1):S51–83.
3. Meaney PA, Bobrow BJ, Mancini ME, et al. CPR quality: improving cardiac resuscitation outcomes both inside and outside the hospital. A consensus statement from the American Heart Association. Circulation 2013;128:417–35.
4. Brooks SC, Anderson ML, Bruder E, et al. Part 6: alternative techniques and ancillary devices for cardiopulmonary resuscitation: 2015 American Heart Association guidelines update for cardiopulmonary resuscitation and emergency cardiovascular care. Circulation 2015;132(18 Suppl 2):S436–43.
5. Buckler DG, Burke RV, Naim MY, et al. Association of mechanical cardiopulmonary resuscitation device use with cardiac arrest outcomes: a population-based study using the CARES registry (cardiac

arrest registry to enhance survival). Circulation 2016;134(25):2131–3.

6. Ong M, Ornato JP, Edwards DP, et al. Use of an automated, load-distributing band chest compression device for out-of-hospital cardiac arrest resuscitation. JAMA 2006;295(22):2629–37.

7. Steen S, Sjoberg T, Olsson P, et al. Treatment of out-of-hospital cardiac arrest with LUCAS, a new device for automatic mechanical compression and active decompression resuscitation. Resuscitation 2005; 67(1):25–30.

8. Axelsson C, Herrera MJ, Fredriksson M, et al. Implementation of mechanical chest compression in out-of-hospital cardiac arrest in an emergency medical service system. Am J Emerg Med 2013;31(8): 1196–200.

9. Esibov A, Banville I, Chapman FW, et al. Mechanical chest compressions improved aspects of CPR in the LINC trial. Resuscitation 2015;91:116–21.

10. Tranberg T, Lassen JF, Kaltoft AK, et al. Quality of cardiopulmonary resuscitation in out-of-hospital cardiac arrest before and after introduction of a mechanical chest compression device, LUCAS-2; a prospective, observational study. Scand J Trauma Resusc Emerg Med 2015;23:37.

11. Yost D, Phillips RH, Gonzales L, et al. Assessment of CPR interruptions from transthoracic impedance during use of the LUCAS™ mechanical chest compression system. Resuscitation 2012;83(8): 961–5.

12. Levy M, Yost D, Walker RG, et al. A quality improvement initiative to optimize use of a mechanical chest compression device within a high-performance CPR approach to out-of-hospital cardiac arrest resuscitation. Resuscitation 2015;92:32–7.

13. Ong ME, Annathurai A, Shahidah A, et al. Cardiopulmonary resuscitation interruptions with use of a load-distributing band device during emergency department cardiac arrest. Ann Emerg Med 2010; 56(3):233–41.

14. Tomte O, Sunde K, Lorem T, et al. Advanced life support performance with manual and mechanical chest compressions in a randomized, multicentre manikin study. Resuscitation 2009;80(10):1152–7.

15. Hallstrom A, Rea TD, Sayre MR, et al. Manual chest compression vs use of an automated chest compression device during resuscitation following out-of-hospital cardiac arrest: a randomized trial. JAMA 2006;295(22):2620–8.

16. Halperin HR, Paradis N, Ornato JP, et al. Cardiopulmonary resuscitation with a novel chest compression device in a porcine model of cardiac arrest: improved hemodynamics and mechanisms. J Am Coll Cardiol 2004;44(11):2214–20.

17. Timerman S, Cardoso LF, Ramires JA, et al. Improved hemodynamic performance with a novel chest compression device during treatment of in-hospital cardiac arrest. Resuscitation 2004; 61(3):273–80.

18. Rubertsson S, Karlsten R. Increased cortical cerebral blood flow with LUCAS; a new device for mechanical chest compressions compared to standard external compressions during experimental cardiopulmonary resuscitation. Resuscitation 2005; 65(3):357–63.

19. Axelsson C, Karlsson T, Axelsson AB, et al. Mechanical active compression-decompression cardiopulmonary resuscitation (ACD-CPR) versus manual CPR according to pressure of end tidal carbon dioxide (P(ET)CO2) during CPR in out-of-hospital cardiac arrest (OHCA). Resuscitation 2009;80(10):1099–103.

20. Dickinson ET, Verdile VP, Schneider RM, et al. Effectiveness of mechanical versus manual chest compressions in out-of-hospital cardiac arrest resuscitation: a pilot study. Am J Emerg Med 1998; 16(3):289–92.

21. Ogawa Y, Shiozaki T, Hirose T, et al. Load-distributing-band cardiopulmonary resuscitation for out-of-hospital cardiac arrest increases regional cerebral oxygenation: a single-center prospective pilot study. Scand J Trauma Resusc Emerg Med 2015; 23:99.

22. Ong ME, Mackey KE, Zhang ZC, et al. Mechanical CPR devices compared to manual CPR during out-of-hospital cardiac arrest and ambulance transport: a systematic review. Scand J Trauma Resusc Emerg Med 2012;20:39.

23. Li H, Wang D, Yu Y, et al. Mechanical versus manual chest compressions for cardiac arrest: a systematic review and meta-analysis. Scand J Trauma Resusc Emerg Med 2016;24:10.

24. Bonnes JL, Brouwer MA, Navarese EP, et al. Manual cardiopulmonary resuscitation versus CPR including a mechanical chest compression device in out-of-hospital cardiac arrest: a comprehensive meta-analysis from randomized and observational studies. Ann Emerg Med 2016;67(3):349–60.e3.

25. Brooks SC, Hassan N, Bigham BL, et al. Mechanical versus manual chest compressions for cardiac arrest. Cochrane Database Syst Rev 2014;(2): CD007260.

26. Gates S, Quinn T, Deakin CD, et al. Mechanical chest compression for out of hospital cardiac arrest: systematic review and meta-analysis. Resuscitation 2015;94:91–7.

27. Smekal D, Johansson J, Huzevka T, et al. A pilot study of mechanical chest compressions with the LUCAS™ device in cardiopulmonary resuscitation. Resuscitation 2011;82(6):702–6.

28. Perkins GD, Lall R, Quinn T, et al. Mechanical versus manual chest compression for out-of-hospital cardiac arrest (PARAMEDIC): a pragmatic, cluster randomised controlled trial. Lancet 2015;385(9972): 947–55.

29. Rubertsson S, Lindgren E, Smekal D, et al. Mechanical chest compressions and simultaneous defibrillation vs conventional cardiopulmonary resuscitation in out-of-hospital cardiac arrest: the linc randomized trial. JAMA 2014;311(1):53–61.

30. Wik L, Olsen J-A, Persse D, et al. Manual vs. integrated automatic load-distributing band CPR with equal survival after out of hospital cardiac arrest. The randomized CIRC trial. Resuscitation 2014; 85(6):741–8.

31. Dyson K, Bray J, Smith K, et al. Paramedic exposure to out-of-hospital cardiac arrest is rare and declining in Victoria, Australia. Resuscitation 2015;89:93–8.

32. Olasveengen TM, Wik L, Steen PA. Quality of cardiopulmonary resuscitation before and during transport in out-of-hospital cardiac arrest. Resuscitation 2008; 76(2):185–90.

33. Stone CK, Thomas SH. Can correct closed-chest compressions be performed during prehospital transport? Prehosp Disaster Med 1995;10(2):121–3.

34. Chung TN, Kim SW, Cho YS, et al. Effect of vehicle speed on the quality of closed-chest compression during ambulance transport. Resuscitation 2016; 81(7):841–7.

35. Sasson C, Hegg AJ, Macy M, et al. Prehospital termination of resuscitation in cases of refractory out-of-hospital cardiac arrest. JAMA 2008;300(12): 1432–8.

36. Morrison LJ, Verbeek PR, Vermeulen MJ, et al. Derivation and evaluation of a termination of resuscitation clinical prediction rule for advanced life support providers. Resuscitation 2007;74(2):266–75.

37. Morrison LJ, Verbeek PR, Zhan C, et al. Validation of a universal prehospital termination of resuscitation clinical prediction rule for advanced and basic life support providers. Resuscitation 2009;80(3):324–8.

38. Morrison LJ, Visentin LM, Kiss A, et al. Validation of a rule for termination of resuscitation in out-of-hospital cardiac arrest. N Engl J Med 2006;355(5):478.

39. Slattery DE, Silver A. The hazards of providing care in emergency vehicles: an opportunity for reform. Prehosp Emerg Care 2009;13(3):388–97.

40. Jones AY, Lee RY. Cardiopulmonary resuscitation and back injury in ambulance officers. Int Arch Occup Environ Health 2005;78(4):332–6.

41. Gassler H, Ventzke MM, Lampl L, et al. Transport with ongoing resuscitation: a comparison between manual and mechanical compression. Emerg Med J 2013;30(7):589–92.

42. Sunde K, Wik L, Steen PA. Quality of mechanical, manual standard and active compression-decompression CPR on the arrest site and during transport in a manikin model. Resuscitation 1997; 34(3):235–42.

43. Stapleton ER. Comparing CPR during ambulance transport. Manual vs. mechanical methods. JEMS 1991;16(9):63–4, 66, 68 passim.

44. Fox J, Fiechter R, Gerstl P, et al. Mechanical versus manual chest compression CPR under ground ambulance transport conditions. Acute Card Care 2013;15(1):1–6.

45. Gassler H, Kummerle S, Ventzke MM, et al. Mechanical chest compression: an alternative in helicopter emergency medical services? Intern Emerg Med 2015;10(6):715–20.

46. Tazarourte K, Sapir D, Laborne FX, et al. Refractory cardiac arrest in a rural area: mechanical chest compression during helicopter transport. Acta Anaesthesiol Scand 2013;57(1):71–6.

47. Hightower D, Thomas SH, Stone CK, et al. Decay in quality of closed-chest compressions over time. Ann Emerg Med 1995;26(3):300–3.

48. Ochoa FJ, Ramalle-Gómara E, Lisa V, et al. The effect of rescuer fatigue on the quality of chest compressions. Resuscitation 1998;37(3):149–52.

49. Hazinski MF, Nolan JP, Aickin R, et al. Part 1: executive summary: 2015 international consensus on cardiopulmonary resuscitation and emergency cardiovascular care science with treatment recommendations. Circulation 2015;132(16 Suppl 1):S2–39.

50. Callaway CW, Donnino MW, Fink EL, et al. Part 8: post-cardiac arrest care: 2015 American Heart Association guidelines update for cardiopulmonary resuscitation and emergency cardiovascular care. Circulation 2015;132(18 Suppl 2):S465–82.

51. Gheeraert PJ, Henriques JPS, De Buyzere ML, et al. Out-of-hospital ventricular fibrillation in patients with acute myocardial infarction: coronary angiographic determinants. J Am Coll Cardiol 2000;35(1):144–50.

52. Sunde K, Pytte M, Jacobsen D, et al. Implementation of a standardised treatment protocol for post resuscitation care after out-of-hospital cardiac arrest. Resuscitation 2007;73(1):29–39.

53. Spaulding CM, Joly LM, Rosenberg A, et al. Immediate coronary angiography in survivors of out-of-hospital cardiac arrest. N Engl J Med 1997;336(23):1629–33.

54. Dumas F, Cariou A, Manzo-Silberman S, et al. Immediate percutaneous coronary intervention is associated with better survival after out-of-hospital cardiac arrest: insights from the PROCAT (Parisian Region Out of hospital Cardiac ArresT) registry. Circ Cardiovasc Interv 2010;3(3):200–7.

55. Fothergill RT, Watson LR, Virdi GK, et al. Survival of resuscitated cardiac arrest patients with ST-elevation myocardial infarction (STEMI) conveyed directly to a Heart Attack Centre by ambulance clinicians. Resuscitation 2014;85(1):96–8.

56. Kern KB. Optimal treatment of patients surviving out-of-hospital cardiac arrest. JACC Cardiovasc Interv 2012;5(6):597–605.

57. Kagawa E, Dote K, Kato M, et al. Should we emergently revascularize occluded coronaries for cardiac arrest?: rapid-response extracorporeal membrane oxygenation and intra-arrest

percutaneous coronary intervention. Circulation 2012;126(13):1605–13.

58. Sunde K. All you need is flow! Resuscitation 2010; 81(4):371–2.

59. Larsen AI, Hjornevik AS, Ellingsen CL, et al. Cardiac arrest with continuous mechanical chest compression during percutaneous coronary intervention. A report on the use of the LUCAS device. Resuscitation 2007;75(3):454–9.

60. Perkins GD, Brace S, Gates S. Mechanical chest-compression devices: current and future roles. Curr Opin Crit Care 2010;16(3):203–10.

61. Forti A, Zilio G, Zanatta P, et al. Full recovery after prolonged cardiac arrest and resuscitation with mechanical chest compression device during helicopter transportation and percutaneous coronary intervention. J Emerg Med 2014;47(6):632–4.

62. Cirillo F, DeRobertis E, Hinkelbein J. Extracorporeal life support for refractory out-of-hospital cardiac arrest in adults. Trends in Anaesthesia and Critical Care 2016;7-8:26–31.

63. Stub D, Bernard S, Pellegrino V, et al. Refractory cardiac arrest treated with mechanical CPR, hypothermia, ECMO and early reperfusion (the CHEER trial). Resuscitation 2015;86:88–94.

64. Ambulance Victoria. Victorian ambulance cardiac arrest registry annual report 2015-2016. 2017 2017.

65. Yannopoulos D, Bartos JA, Raveendran G, et al. Coronary artery disease in patients with out-of-hospital refractory ventricular fibrillation cardiac arrest. J Am Coll Cardiol 2017;70(9):1109–17.

66. Fagnoul D, Taccone FS, Belhaj A, et al. Extracorporeal life support associated with hypothermia and normoxemia in refractory cardiac arrest. Resuscitation 2013;84(11):1519–24.

67. Yannopoulos D, Bartos JA, Martin C, et al. Minnesota resuscitation consortium's advanced perfusion and reperfusion cardiac life support strategy for out-of-hospital refractory ventricular fibrillation. J Am Heart Assoc 2016;5(6) [pii:e003732].

68. Wik L, Kiil S. Use of an automatic mechanical chest compression device (LUCAS) as a bridge to establishing cardiopulmonary bypass for a patient with hypothermic cardiac arrest. Resuscitation 2005; 66(3):391–4.

69. Holmström P, Boyd J, Sorsa M, et al. A case of hypothermic cardiac arrest treated with an external chest compression device (LUCAS) during transport to rewarming. Resuscitation 2005;67(1):139–41.

70. Friberg H, Rundgren M. Submersion, accidental hypothermia and cardiac arrest, mechanical chest compressions as a bridge to final treatment: a case report. Scand J Trauma Resusc Emerg Med 2009;17:7.

71. Chenaitia H, Fournier M, Brun JP, et al. Association of mechanical chest compression and prehospital thrombolysis. Am J Emerg Med 2012;30(6):1015.e1-2.

Manual Versus Mechanical Cardiopulmonary Resuscitation
A Case Against the Machine

Claire A. Nordeen, MD

KEYWORDS

- Mechanical • Device • Manual • Compression • CPR • Quality • Survival

KEY POINTS

- Mechanical compression devices produce promising results with improved markers of perfusion in animal studies, but these do not translate to human survival.
- There are conflicting data on whether mechanical chest compression devices perform high-quality cardiopulmonary resuscitation (CPR), including compression rate, depth, and fraction, more reliably than humans.
- Mechanical CPR is associated with more traumatic injuries to patients, but these injuries are unlikely to have clinical significance.
- Ongoing CPR during transportation is unsafe for providers, but there is no evidence that mechanical chest compression devices improve its safety profile.
- In large, randomized, prospective, human trials, mechanical CPR is associated with equivalent survival and worse neuro-favorable outcomes when compared with manual CPR.

INTRODUCTION

Resuscitation science and practice made incredible advancements over the past 30 years. At the same time, progress in portable machine technology led to improved consistency, efficiency, and quality in an array of fields, and was thus integrated widely. By 2005, consensus among international leaders in resuscitation advised that chest compressions be performed hard and fast with minimal interruptions.[1] It follows that a mechanized compression device would be capable of delivering such high-performance cardiopulmonary resuscitation (HPCPR)[a] more predictably and reliably than humans, thereby meeting recommended standards and ultimately improving outcomes. Although randomized controlled trials (RCTs) in animal models consistently show favorable outcomes among physiologic markers of perfusion, and both manikin and some human studies have demonstrated superior ability to perform HPCPR with mechanical versus manual chest compressions, large RCTs of out-of-hospital cardiac arrest (OHCA) have failed to show a survival advantage. Furthermore, these

Disclosure Statement: The author receives a portion of fellowship funding through a grant from Physio-Control.

Department of Emergency Medicine, University of Washington, Harborview Medical Center, Box 359727, 325 9th Avenue, Seattle, WA 98122, USA

E-mail address: cnordeen@uw.edu

[a] Or *high-quality CPR* refers to CPR that meets recommended standards for rate (100–120), depth (5–6 cm), fraction (>0.8), and peri-shock pause (<10 seconds); limits pauses in general; allows for chest wall recoil.

Cardiol Clin 36 (2018) 375–386
https://doi.org/10.1016/j.ccl.2018.03.005

Nordeen

trials have trended toward worse neurologic outcomes among patients treated with mechanical chest compression devices. Despite years of research efforts trying to convince ourselves otherwise, available evidence cannot support the widespread use of mechanical chest compression devices, at least in their current form.

Several key assumptions comprise the argument supporting the use of mechanical chest compression devices in OHCA:

- High-quality cardiopulmonary resuscitation (CPR) is associated with better outcomes in cardiac arrest.

- There is wide variability in and degradation of chest compression performance during manual CPR, especially during patient extrication and transport to the hospital.
- Mechanical devices are able to achieve more consistent, high-quality CPR than manual compressions, *and* this holds true in the prehospital environment.
- Consistency in CPR is desirable.
- Mechanical devices are safer (associated with fewer adverse effects) for both providers and patients.

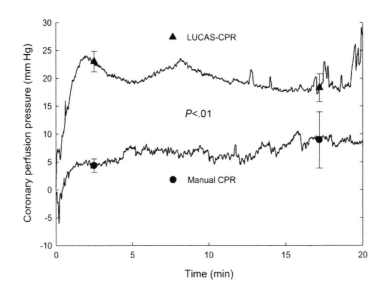

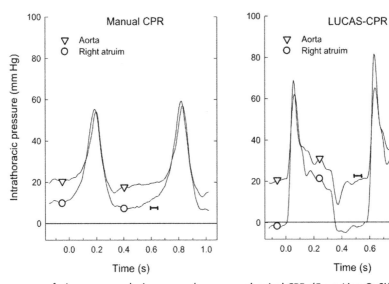

Fig. 1. Coronary perfusion pressure during manual versus mechanical CPR. (*From* Liao Q, Sjöberg T, Paskevicius A, et al. Manual versus mechanical cardiopulmonary resuscitation. An experimental study in pigs. BMC Cardio Dis 2010;10(1):4; with permission.)

The following sections explore the evidence behind each of these statements.

Consistent, High-Quality Cardiopulmonary Resuscitation Is Associated with Better Outcomes in Cardiac Arrest

According to the American Heart Association (AHA), "high quality CPR is the cornerstone of a system of care that can optimize outcomes beyond return of spontaneous circulation."[2] Systems in which the cardiac arrest Chain of Survival (of which early HPCPR plays a large part) is effectively implemented can achieve witnessed ventricular fibrillation cardiac arrest survival approaching 50%, far surpassing the rates in systems with missing links in this chain.[3] In 2006, one observational trial showed that increased compression depth and decreased preshock pauses in CPR were associated with defibrillation success,[4] whereas another group demonstrated that increasing the chest compression fraction by decreasing peri-shock pauses correlated directly with survival.[5] More recently, Cheskes and colleagues[6] examined the association between compliance with the AHA's increasingly ambitious CPR quality guidelines and patient outcomes, demonstrating that adherence to HPCPR was associated with a 2-fold increase in survival to hospital discharge and a 3-fold increase in neuro-favorable survival among patients with prolonged (>10 minutes) resuscitation.

Mechanical Cardiopulmonary Resuscitation Is Associated with Improved Markers of Perfusion but Not Survival

Animal models investigating the effects of mechanical versus manual CPR on hemodynamic variables show promising evidence in favor of mechanical devices, some of which have been replicated in humans. Wik and colleagues[7] randomized dogs to manual versus mechanical compressions and found that central arterial pressure and coronary perfusion pressure were higher among the device group, though there was no difference in survival. A later pig model corroborated these findings (**Fig. 1**) in addition to showing significantly higher end-tidal carbon dioxide (CO_2), carotid blood flow (**Fig. 2**), and rate of return of spontaneous circulation (ROSC) among the mechanical CPR group.[8] Such invasive methods of exact hemodynamic monitoring are generally not feasible in human studies of OHCA. Two randomized trials comparing mechanical with manual CPR found higher, sustained end-tidal CO_2 levels in the mechanical arm[9,10]; neither were associated with survival.

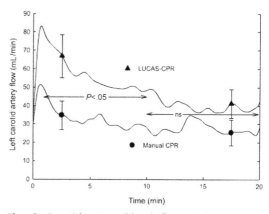

Fig. 2. Carotid artery blood flow during manual versus mechanical CPR. (*From* Liao Q, Sjöberg T, Paskevicius A, et al. Manual versus mechanical cardiopulmonary resuscitation. An experimental study in pigs. BMC Cardio Dis 2010;10(1):5; with permission.)

Human Factors Associated with the Use of Mechanical Compression Devices May Contribute to, but Cannot Fully Account for, Conflicting Data in Its Ability to Improve Cardiopulmonary Resuscitation Quality

Although some evidence supports improved CPR quality with mechanical devices, other data show equivalent or worse outcomes compared with manual. In general, benefits gained from high-quality compressions with the device in place are offset by the time it takes to place the device correctly.

Several manikin studies show higher quality with mechanical CPR compared with manual as measured by outcomes including rate, depth, overall compression fraction, or correct compression fraction.[11-15] Higher compression fraction and rates were corroborated in a handful of human studies as well.[11,16,17]

On the other hand, several manikin and human studies demonstrate equivalent or worse quality with mechanical CPR compared with manual. Although the quality of mechanical CPR can be better once the device is properly situated, the pauses in CPR for device application and deconstruction often increase hands-off time enough to nullify the quality benefits[11,18] (**Fig. 3**). In some cases, device use is associated with significant and unacceptable delays to first defibrillation.[1,3,19,20] Malpositioned devices also lead to inadequate rate and depth of CPR[21] (**Fig. 4**). Newer devices show low rates of error/need for trouble-shooting in randomized human trials,[22] and targeted quality-improvement measures can be successful in minimizing pauses associated

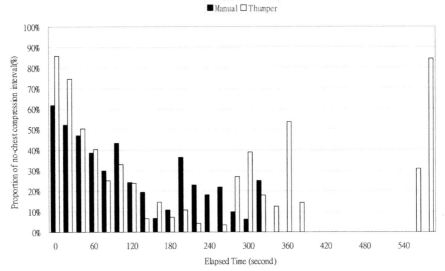

Fig. 3. Proportion of hands-off time per interval of elapsed time during resuscitation. (*From* Wang HC, Chiang WC, Chen SY, et al. Video-recording and time-motion analyses of manual versus mechanical cardiopulmonary resuscitation during ambulance transport. Resuscitation 2007;74(3):457; with permission.)

with device deployment[23]; nevertheless, chest compression fraction and other quality markers are not reliably superior.[22,24,25]

Given that the AHA's guidelines emphasize the importance of decreasing time to defibrillation and pauses around defibrillation,[26] one theoretic advantage held by the mechanical devices is the ability to deliver electricity with ongoing compressions. The algorithm for the prospective, randomized LUCAS in Cardiac Arrest (LINC) trial in humans incorporated this concept, delivering shocks to the mechanical arm in the absence of

rhythm check and while continuing compressions. Although peri-shock pauses were, thus, absent from the mechanical arm, this high-quality performance measure was not associated with increased conversion of shockable to organized rhythm or decreased rates of refibrillation[27] (**Fig. 5**).

Patient Extrication and Transport Make High-Quality Cardiopulmonary Resuscitation Difficult: Mechanical Cardiopulmonary Resuscitation Does Not Perform Better Than Manual Cardiopulmonary Resuscitation Even Under These Specific Circumstances

For obvious reasons, it is difficult to perform high-quality chest compressions while extricating and transporting patients from the scene of arrest to the hospital. Both mathematical modeling of ambulance acceleration vectors[28] and manikin studies suggest that manual CPR quality deteriorates during transportation in a ground ambulance[29] (**Fig. 6**). With increasing availability of hospital-based interventions (percutaneous coronary intervention, invasive rewarming, extracorporeal membrane oxygenation) that may help improve rates of ROSC and survival, depending on the cause of arrest, maintaining high-quality CPR during patient relocation is critical.

Several manikin studies compared manual with mechanical CPR under simulated extrication and transportation scenarios. In a ground transport simulation, paramedic students were unable to generate adequate rate or depth of chest

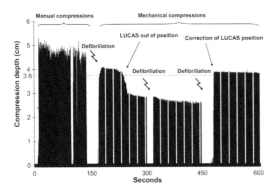

Fig. 4. Effect of device positioning on compression depth in a case of mechanical CPR on a manikin. (*From* Blomberg H, Gedeborg R, Berglund L, et al. Poor chest compression quality with mechanical compressions in simulated cardiopulmonary resuscitation: a randomized, cross-over manikin study. Resuscitation 2011;82(10):1333; with permission.)

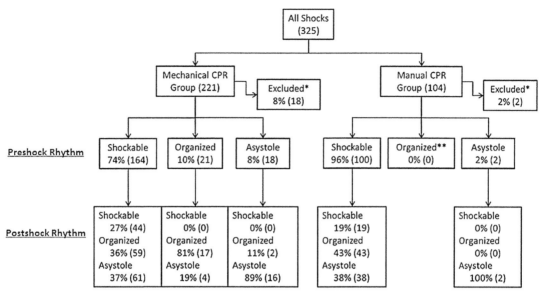

Fig. 5. Outcomes after shock delivery in conventional manual CPR versus mechanical CPR with blind shock application during ongoing compressions. * Annotators unable to determine underlying rhythm. ** No shocks delivered in manual group due to organized rhythm. (*From* Esibov A, Banville I, Chapman FW, et al. Mechanical chest compressions improved aspects of CPR in the LINC trial. Resuscitation 2015;91:119; with permission.)

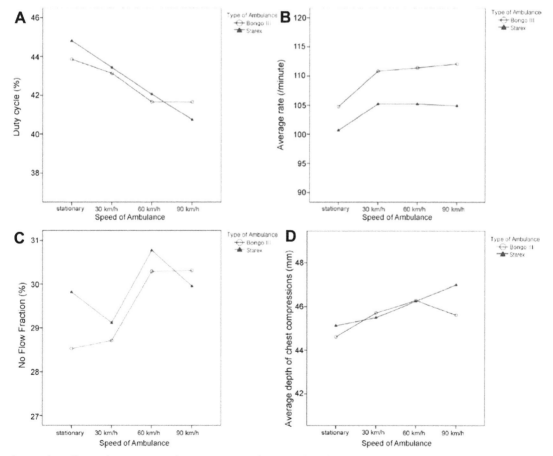

Fig. 6. The effects of varying speeds on measures of CPR quality during manikin simulated transport, including (*A*) duty cycle of chest compressions (%), (*B*) average rate of chest compressions, (*C*) no-flow fraction (%), and (*D*) average depth of chest compressions (mm). (*From* Chung TN, Kim SW, Cho YS, et al. Effect of vehicle speed on the quality of closed-chest compression during ambulance transport. Resuscitation 2010;81(7):845; with permission.)

compressions during transport on a stretcher and in the rig, whereas the mechanical device performed high-quality CPR in both.[30] In a helicopter rescue simulation, mechanical CPR showed better fraction of correct overall compressions, depth, pressure point, and pressure release than manual CPR[13] (**Fig. 7**). In a creative high-rise elevator extrication simulation out of Korea, the use of a mechanical compression device demonstrated lower no-flow fraction during extrication compared with manual CPR when no differences were detected earlier in the stationary on-scene portion of the resuscitation[31] (**Fig. 8**).

No human studies prospectively compare manual and mechanical chest compressions specifically during extrication and transport. A retrospective study of manual CPR in OHCA showed that although compression depth, rate, fraction, and frequency were all worse among transported patients, there was no significant deterioration during transportation.[32] A retrospective before-after study found that overall no-flow time decreased primarily because of CPR continuation during extrication after a

mechanical CPR device was introduced to the system.[33] Finally, a large observational trial showed that prehospital providers could perform manual CPR simultaneously compliant with all 3 of the AHA's recommended 2010 guidelines (rate, depth, compression fraction) for more than 50% of the total resuscitation time, with no significant differences between scene, egress, and transport.[34]

Mechanical Cardiopulmonary Resuscitation Decreases the Variability Seen in Manual Cardiopulmonary Resuscitation, but Machine-Grade Consistency in Chest Compressions May Not Be Beneficial

Manikin studies demonstrate that mechanical devices perform compressions with lower variability of rate and depth compared with manual CPR[15,18,35,36] (**Fig. 9**). A recent RCT in pigs, however, investigates the concept that variability in chest compression rates may actually be beneficial.[37] All pigs were treated with mechanical CPR but were randomized to receive CPR at a consistent rate of 100 per minute versus

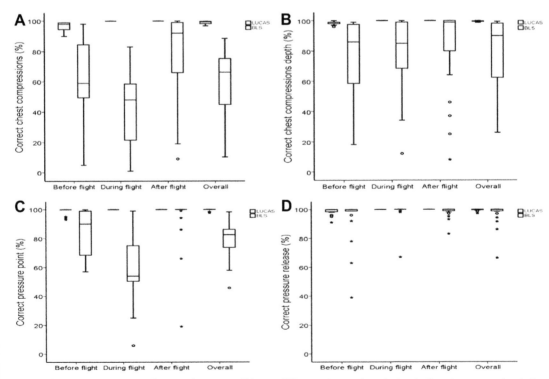

Fig. 7. Chest compression quality metrics on manikins at different time points during helicopter rescue simulation using basic life support (BLS, ie, manual) versus mechanical CPR. Quality metrics compared include (*A*) correct compression fraction (%), (*B*) correct compression depth fraction (%), (*C*) correct CPR pressure point (%), (*D*) correct compression pressure (%). (*From* Putzer G, Braun P, Zimmermann A, et al. LUCAS compared to manual cardiopulmonary resuscitation is more effective during helicopter rescue—a prospective, randomized, cross-over manikin study. Am J Emerg Med 2013;31(2):388; with permission.)

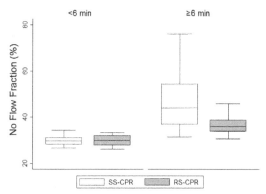

Fig. 8. Hands-off fraction using manual versus mechanical CPR before and during simulated elevator extrication in a manikin resuscitation simulation. SS-CPR, manual CPR on standard stretcher; RS-CPR, mechanical CPR on reducible stretcher. (*From* Kim TH, Hong KJ, Sang Do S, et al. Quality between mechanical compression on reducible stretcher versus manual compression on standard stretcher in small elevator. Am J Emerg Med 2016;34(8):1608; with permission.)

alternating every 6 seconds between rates of 100 and 200 per minute, mimicking human error. The time-varying group achieved higher cerebral perfusion pressure, pulmonary artery oxygen saturation, end-tidal CO_2, and rate of ROSC at 5 minutes (**Fig. 10**), suggesting that human erraticism may inform compression device design in a way that ultimately improves outcomes.

Mechanical Cardiopulmonary Resuscitation Is Associated with More Traumatic Injuries to Patients, but These Are Unlikely to Affect Outcome

According to autopsy data, the use of mechanical CPR devices is associated with a 3-fold risk of any injury and a 2-fold risk of rib fracture. There is no evidence that these injuries are clinically relevant to ultimate survival outcome,[38] and their contribution to the patients' course during rehabilitation among survivors has not been examined.

Ongoing Cardiopulmonary Resuscitation During Transportation Is Unsafe for Providers, but There Is No Evidence That Mechanical Chest Compression Devices Improve Its Safety Profile

Crashes are a common occurrence within the working life span of emergency medical services (EMS) providers, and the most serious work-related injuries suffered by EMS providers are crash related.[39] Rear-seat occupancy and lack of restraint use are independently associated with a risk of serious or fatal injury in the event of a crash, with odds ratios (ORs) of 2.7 and 2.5, respectively.[40] Use of lights and sirens increases the incidence of crashing in general, in addition to injury after crash.[39,41] Given that transportation of patients with ongoing manual CPR generally requires providers to be unbelted in the back of an ambulance driving with lights and sirens, it may be "hazardous to the personnel and was suggested [to be] unethical."[16] The World Health Organization reports that among rear-seat occupants, seat belts reduce fatal and serious injuries by 25% and minor injuries by 75%.[42] In theory, mechanical CPR devices could reduce injuries by allowing providers to remain restrained during transport despite ongoing chest compressions. This theory assumes, however, that chest compressions are the only component requiring providers to be mobile during the complicated care of

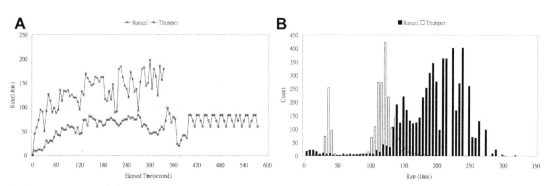

Fig. 9. Comparison of chest compression rate between manual and mechanical CPR during transport. (*A*) Comparison of chest compression rate during transport. (*B*) Comparison of distributions of chest compression rate by minute during transport. (*From* Wang HC, Chiang WC, Chen SY, et al. Video-recording and time-motion analyses of manual versus mechanical cardiopulmonary resuscitation during ambulance transport. Resuscitation 2007;74(3):456; with permission.)

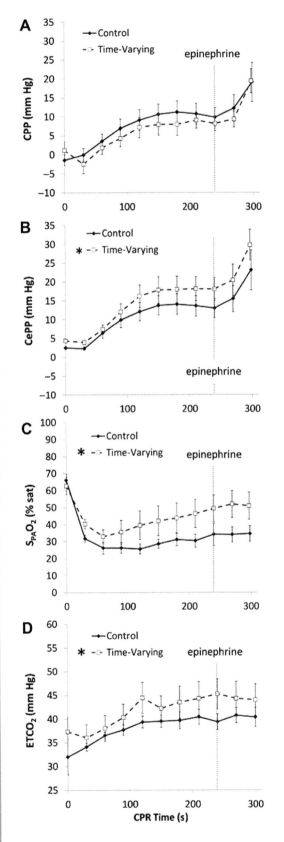

pulseless patients. Moreover, the independent risk factors associated with rear-seat occupancy and driving under emergent conditions will remain unaffected by this change. For a population of patients whose survival is only 5% to 6%[32] (ie, those transported without ROSC), mandating EMS providers to undertake this risk without evidence that mechanical CPR actually reduces the risk of injury is ethically questionable.

The Case Against Mechanical Cardiopulmonary Resuscitation: in Theory It Should Work, in Practice It Does Not

Despite promising data on perfusion in animal models and some CPR quality metrics in manikins and humans, the case for mechanical compression devices ultimately fails because it lacks support on the grounds of real-world application and patient-centered outcomes. The end goal of resuscitation is not to have a higher end-tidal CO_2 or achieve a perfect chest compression fraction but to restore a meaningful quality of life to patients after cardiac arrest. Of the large, prospective, human RCTs on this topic, none demonstrated improved cardiac arrest survival (including at 4 hours, 1 month, and 6 months) among patients receiving mechanical CPR[20,22,24] (**Table 1**). Of greater concern, a subgroup analysis in one of these trials showed a *lower* 30-day survival rate among patients with initially shockable rhythms (OR 0.71, 95% confidence interval [CI] 0.52–0.98).[43] Several reviews and meta-analyses have been performed on this topic; none have rejected the null hypothesis[12,43,44] (**Table 2**).

A handful of studies comparing manual with mechanical CPR have found that mechanical CPR is associated with worse neurologic outcomes among cardiac arrest survivors.[16,20,25,43–45] In 2006, the ASPIRE (AutoPulse Assisted Prehospital International Resuscitation) trial was terminated early after safety review because of significantly worse Cerebral Performance Scores among patients in the mechanical

Fig. 10. Markers of perfusion initial 5 minutes of CPR in a pig model comparing standard and time-varying approaches with mechanical CPR and comparing differences in (*A*) coronary perfusion pressure (CPP), (*B*) cerebral perfusion pressure (CePP), (*C*) pulmonary arterial oxygen saturation ($S_{PA}O_2$), (*D*) end tidal CO_2 (ETCO$_2$). (*From* Taylor TG, Esibov A, Melnick SB, et al. Will alternating between fast and slow chest compressions improve resuscitation outcomes? Circulation 2017;136:A16908; with permission.)

Table 1
Survival and neurologic status among patients with cardiac arrest treated with mechanical versus manual cardiopulmonary resuscitation

Outcomes	No. of Participants (%)			Treatment Difference (%) (95% CI)
	Mechanical CPR (n = 1300)	Manual CPR (n = 1289)	P Value	
4-h survival[a]	307 (23.6)	305 (23.7)	>.99	−0.05 (−3.3–3.2)
ROSC[b]	460 (35.4)	446 (34.6)	.68	0.78 (−2.9–4.5)
Arrival at emergency department with palpable pulse	366 (28.2)	357 (27.7)	.83	0.46 (−3.0–3.9)
Survival to discharge from ICU with CPC 1–2[c]	98 (7.5)	82 (6.4)	.25	1.18 (−0.8–3.1)
Survival to hospital discharge with CPC 1–2[c]	108 (8.3)	100 (7.8)	.61	0.55 (−1.5–2.6)
1-mo survival with CPC I-2[d]	105 (8.1)	94 (7.3)	.46	0.78 (−1.3–2.8)
6-mo survival with CPC I-2[d]	110 (8.5)	98 (7.6)	.43	0.86 (−1.2–3.0)
Survival to discharge from ICU[e]	158 (12.2)	153 (11.9)	.86	0.28 (−2.2–2.8)
With CPC 1	54 (4.2)	34 (2.6)	.04	1.52 (0.1–2.9)
With CPC 2	44 (3.4)	48 (3.7)	—	—
With CPC 3	34 (2.6)	40 (3.1)	—	—
With CPC 4	26 (2.0)	29 (2.2)	—	—
Survival to discharge from hospital[e]	117 (9.0)	118 (9.2)	.89	−0.15 (−2.4–2.1)
With CPC 1	89 (6.8)	67 (5.2)	.08	1.65 (−0.2–3.5)
With CPC 2	19 (1.5)	33 (2.6)	—	—
With CPC 3	9 (0.7)	15 (1.2)	—	—
With CPC 4	0	1 (0.1)	—	—
1-mo survival[f]	112 (8.6)	109 (8.5)	.89	0.16 (−2.0–2.3)
With CPC 1	92 (7.1)	74 (5.7)	.17	1.34 (−0.6–3.2)
With CPC 2	13 (1.0)	20 (1.6)	—	—
With CPC 3	7 (0.5)	13 (1.0)	—	—
With CPC 4	0	1 (0.1)	—	—
6-mo survival[g]	111 (8.5)	104 (8.1)	.67	0.47 (−1.7–2.6)
With CPC 1	103 (7.9)	88 (6.8)	.29	1.10 (−0.9–3.1)
With CPC 2	7 (0.5)	10 (0.8)	—	—
With CPC 3	1 (0.1)	6 (0.5)	—	—
With CPC 4	0	0	—	—

Abbreviations: CPC, cerebral performance category score; ICU, intensive care unit.
[a] One patient in mechanical CPR group and 3 in manual CPR group with unknown 4-hour survival were imputed as nonsurvivors.
[b] Two patients in mechanical CPR group and 1 in manual CPR group with unknown ROSC were imputed as having no ROSC.
[c] Ten patients in mechanical CPR group and 8 in manual CPR group with unknown outcome were imputed as having a bad outcome.
[d] Fourteen patients in mechanical CPR group and 15 in manual CPR group with unknown outcome were imputed as having a bad outcome.
[e] Ten patients in mechanical CPR group and 6 in manual CPR group with unknown outcome were imputed as nonsurvivors.
[f] Fourteen patients in mechanical CPR group and 14 in manual CPR group with unknown outcome were imputed as nonsurvivors.
[g] Fourteen patients in mechanical CPR group and 15 in manual CPR group with unknown outcome were imputed as nonsurvivors.
From Rubertsson S, Lindgren E, Smekal D, et al. Mechanical chest compressions and simultaneous defibrillation vs conventional cardiopulmonary resuscitation in out-of-hospital cardiac arrest: the LINC randomized trial JAMA 2014;311(1):58; with permission.

Table 2
Odds ratio relating to survival in a meta-analysis of prospective, randomized human trials comparing manual with mechanical cardiopulmonary resuscitation

Study or Subgroup	log[Odds Ratio]	SE	Weight	Odds Ratio IV, Random, 95% CI
1.3.1 LUCAS				
Smekal 2011	-0.2139	0.5826	1.5%	0.81 [0.26, 2.53]
PARAMEDIC	-0.1508	0.1507	22.7%	0.86 [0.64, 1.16]
LINC	0.0203	0.1408	26.0%	1.02 [0.77, 1.34]
Subtotal (95% CI)			50.2%	0.94 [0.77, 1.14]
Heterogeneity: Tau² = 0.00; Chi² = 0.76, df = 2 (P = .69); I² = 0%				
Test for overall effect: Z = 0.63 (P = .53)				
1.3.2 Autopulse				
CIRC	-0.1165	0.1082	44.0%	0.89 [0.72, 1.10]
ASPIRE	-0.5798	0.3001	5.7%	0.56 [0.31, 1.01]
Subtotal (95% CI)			49.8%	0.77 [0.50, 1.17]
Heterogeneity: Tau² = 0.06; Chi² = 2.11, df = 1 (P = .15); I² = 53%				
Test for overall effect: Z = 1.22 (P = .22)				
Total (95% CI)			100.0%	0.89 [0.77, 1.02]
Heterogeneity: Tau² = 0.00; Chi² = 3.41, df = 4 (P = .49); I² = 0%				
Test for overall effect: Z = 1.63 (P = .10)				
Test for subgroup differences: Chi² = 0.70, df = 1 (P = .40), I² = 0%				

Favours manual Favours mechanical (0.1 0.2 0.5 1 2 5 10)

From Gates S, Quinn T, Deakin CD, et al. Mechanical chest compression for out of hospital cardiac arrest: systematic review and meta-analysis. Resuscitation 2015;94:95; with permission.

arm.[20] In the PARAMEDIC (Mechanical versus manual chest compression for out-of-hospital cardiac arrest) trial, the adjusted OR for a neuro-favorable outcome in the mechanical group was 0.72 (95% CI 0.52–0.99).[43] Youngquist and colleagues[45] corroborated these findings in a retrospective study using propensity score analysis (**Table 3**).

SUMMARY

Why this device that holds so much promise fails to perform as expected in the real world is not totally clear. Perhaps there is something unquantifiable, even ethereal, in the application of human touch during CPR that affects outcomes in cardiac arrest, snatching life from the jaws of death. So-called touch therapy is a cornerstone of traditional healing; its application to allopathic medicine is rapidly growing, yielding beneficial effects, such as accelerated growth in premature babies, lowered glucose levels in children with diabetes, reduction in pain perception, improved immune response in patients with cancer, and improved wound healing.[46] Whatever the underlying mechanism, mechanical CPR devices provide a solution to which the specific problem has yet to be identified. They may yet have a role to play in a certain patient population, at a certain time, and in a certain situation; but that role begs definition. In a world with limited resources, this costly one cannot yet justify its place.

Table 3
Odds of neuro-intact survival after resuscitation with manual versus mechanical cardiopulmonary resuscitation

	Relative Risk	(95% CI)	P value
All cases	0.41	(0.24–0.70)	.001
By initial rhythm			
Shockable	0.47	(0.25–0.86)	.015
Asystole	0.41	(0.11–1.57)	.194
PEA	0.24	(0.02–2.26)	.211
EMS witnessed	0.18	(0.08–0.40)	<.0001
Early field ROSC excluded	0.53	(0.29–1.0)	.05
Auto-pulse only	0.51	(0.28–0.94)	.028

Abbreviations: PEA, pulseless electrical activity; ROSC, return of spontaneous circulation.
From Youngquist ST, Ockerse P, Hartsell S, et al. Mechanical chest compression devices are associated with poor neurological survival in a statewide registry: a propensity score analysis. Resuscitation 2016;106:106; with permission.

REFERENCES

1. International Liaison Committee on Resuscitation. 2005 international consensus on cardiopulmonary resuscitation and emergency cardiovascular care science with treatment recommendations. Part 2:

adult basic life support. Resuscitation 2005;67(2–3):187–201.

2. Field J, Hazinski MF, Sayre MR, et al. Part 1: executive summary 2010 American Heart Association guidelines for cardiopulmonary resuscitation and emergency cardiovascular care. Circulation 2010; 122(18):S640–56.

3. Travers AH, Rea TD, Bobrow BJ, et al. Part 4: CPR overview: 2010 American Heart Association guidelines for cardiopulmonary resuscitation and emergency cardiovascular care. Circulation 2010; 122(18 Suppl 3):S676–84.

4. Edelson DP, Abella BS, Kramer-Johanson J, et al. Effects of compression depth and pre-shock pauses predict defibrillation failure during cardiac arrest. Resuscitation 2006;71(2):137–45.

5. Rea TD, Helbock M, Perry S, et al. Increasing use of cardiopulmonary resuscitation during out-of-hospital ventricular fibrillation arrest: survival implications of guideline changes. Circulation 2006;114(25):2760–5.

6. Cheskes S, Schmicker RH, Rea T, et al. The association between AHA CPR quality guideline compliance and clinical outcomes from out-of-hospital cardiac arrest. Resuscitation 2017;116:39–45.

7. Wik L, Bircher NG, Safar P. A comparison of prolonged manual and mechanical external chest compression after cardiac arrest in dogs. Resuscitation 1996;32(3):241–50.

8. Liao Q, Sjöberg T, Paskevicius A, et al. Manual versus mechanical cardiopulmonary resuscitation. An experimental study in pigs. BMC Cardiovasc Disord 2010;10(1):1–8.

9. Dickinson ET, Verdile VP, Schneider RM, et al. Effectiveness of mechanical versus manual chest compressions in out-of-hospital cardiac arrest resuscitation: a pilot study. Am J Emerg Med 1998; 16(3):289–92.

10. Axelsson C, Herrera MJ, Fredriksson M, et al. Implementation of mechanical chest compression in out-of-hospital cardiac arrest in an emergency medical service system. Am J Emerg Med 2013;31(8): 1196–200.

11. Yost D, Phillips RH, Gonzales L, et al. Assessment of CPR interruptions from transthoracic impedance during use of the LUCAS™ mechanical chest compression system. Resuscitation 2012;83(8): 961–5.

12. Ong ME, Mackey KE, Zhang ZC, et al. Mechanical CPR devices compared to manual CPR during out-of-hospital cardiac arrest and ambulance transport: a systematic review. Scand J Trauma Resusc Emerg Med 2012;20(1):1–10.

13. Putzer G, Braun P, Zimmermann A, et al. LUCAS compared to manual cardiopulmonary resuscitation is more effective during helicopter rescue—a prospective, randomized, cross-over manikin study. Am J Emerg Med 2013;31(2):384–9.

14. Putzer G, Fiala A, Braun P, et al. Manual versus mechanical chest compressions on surfaces of varying softness with or without backboards: a randomized, crossover manikin study. J Emerg Med 2016;50(4): 594–600.

15. Gässler H, Ventzke MM, Lampl L, et al. Transport with ongoing resuscitation: a comparison between manual and mechanical compression. Emerg Med J 2012;30(7):589–92.

16. Olasveengen TM, Wik L, Steen PA. Quality of cardiopulmonary resuscitation before and during transport in out-of-hospital cardiac arrest. Resuscitation 2008; 76(2):185–90.

17. Tranberg T, Lassen JF, Kaltoft AK, et al. Quality of cardiopulmonary resuscitation in out-of-hospital cardiac arrest before and after introduction of a mechanical chest compression device, LUCAS-2; a prospective, observational study. Scand J Trauma Resusc Emerg Med 2015;23(1):1–8.

18. Wang HC, Chiang WC, Chen SY, et al. Videorecording and time-motion analyses of manual versus mechanical cardiopulmonary resuscitation during ambulance transport. Resuscitation 2007; 74(3):453–60.

19. Tomte O, Sunde K, Lorem T, et al. Advanced life support performance with manual and mechanical chest compressions in a randomized, multicentre manikin study. Resuscitation 2009;80(10): 1152–7.

20. Hallstrom A, Rea TD, Sayre MR, et al. Manual chest compression vs use of an automated chest compression device during resuscitation following out-of-hospital cardiac arrest: a randomized trial. JAMA 2006;295(22):2620–8.

21. Blomberg H, Gedeborg R, Berglund L, et al. Poor chest compression quality with mechanical compressions in simulated cardiopulmonary resuscitation: a randomized, cross-over manikin study. Resuscitation 2011;82(10):1332–7.

22. Rubertsson S, Lindgren E, Smekal D, et al. Mechanical chest compressions and simultaneous defibrillation vs conventional cardiopulmonary resuscitation in out-of-hospital cardiac arrest: the LINC randomized trial. JAMA 2014;311(1):53–61.

23. Levy M, Yost D, Walker RG, et al. A quality improvement initiative to optimize use of a mechanical chest compression device within a high-performance CPR approach to out-of-hospital cardiac arrest resuscitation. Resuscitation 2015;92:32–7.

24. Wik L, Olsen JA, Persse D, et al. Manual vs. integrated automatic load-distributing band CPR with equal survival after out of hospital cardiac arrest. The randomized CIRC trial. Resuscitation 2014; 85(6):741–8.

25. Zeiner S, Sulzgruber P, Datler P, et al. Mechanical chest compression does not seem to improve outcome after out-of-hospital cardiac arrest. A single

center observational trial. Resuscitation 2015;96:
220–5.

26. Neumar RW, Shuster M, Callaway CW, et al. Executive summary: 2015 American Heart Association guidelines update for cardiopulmonary resuscitation and emergency cardiovascular care. Circulation 2015;132(18 Suppl 2):S315–67.

27. Esibov A, Banville I, Chapman FW, et al. Mechanical chest compressions improved aspects of CPR in the LINC trial. Resuscitation 2015;91:116–21.

28. Kurz MC, Dante SA, Puckett BJ. Estimating the impact of off-balancing forces upon cardiopulmonary resuscitation during ambulance transport. Resuscitation 2012;83(9):1085–9.

29. Chung TN, Kim SW, Cho YS, et al. Effect of vehicle speed on the quality of closed-chest compression during ambulance transport. Resuscitation 2010; 81(7):841–7.

30. Sunde K, Wik L, Steen PA. Quality of mechanical, manual standard and active compression-decompression CPR on the arrest site and during transport in a manikin model. Resuscitation 1997; 34(3):235–42.

31. Kim TH, Hong KJ, Sang Do S, et al. Quality between mechanical compression on reducible stretcher versus manual compression on standard stretcher in small elevator. Am J Emerg Med 2016;34(8): 1604–9.

32. Ødegaard S, Olasveengen T, Steen PA, et al. The effect of transport on quality of cardiopulmonary resuscitation in out-of-hospital cardiac arrest. Resuscitation 2009;80(8):843–8.

33. Lyon RM, Crawford A, Crookston C, et al. The combined use of mechanical CPR and a carry sheet to maintain quality resuscitation in out-of-hospital cardiac arrest patients during extrication and transport. Resuscitation 2015;93:102–6.

34. Cheskes S, Byers A, Zhan C, et al. CPR quality during out-of-hospital cardiac arrest transport. Resuscitation 2017;114:34–9.

35. Roosa JR, Vadeboncoeur TF, Dommer PB, et al. CPR variability during ground ambulance transport of patients in cardiac arrest. Resuscitation 2013; 84(5):592–5.

36. Fox J, Fiechter R, Gerstl P, et al. Mechanical versus manual chest compression CPR underground ambulance transport conditions. Acute Card Care 2013;15(1):1–6.

37. Taylor TG, Esibov A, Melnick SB, et al. Will alternating between fast and slow chest compressions improve resuscitation outcomes? Circulation 2017; 136:A16908.

38. Smekal D, Johansson J, Huzevka T, et al. A pilot study of mechanical chest compressions with the LUCAS™ device in cardiopulmonary resuscitation. Resuscitation 2011;82(6):702–6.

39. Becker LR, Zaloshnja E, Levick N, et al. Relative risk of injury and death in ambulances and other emergency vehicles. Accid Anal Prev 2003;35(6):941–8.

40. Kahn CA, Pirrallo RG, Kuhn EM. Characteristics of fatal ambulance crashes in the United States: an 11-year retrospective analysis. Prehosp Emerg Care 2001;5(3):261–9.

41. Saunders CE, Heye CJ. Ambulance collisions in an urban environment. Prehosp Disaster Med 1994; 9(2):118–24.

42. WHO Library Cataloguing-in-Publication Data. Global status report on road safety. WHO; 2015.

43. Brooks SC, Hassan N, Bigham BL, et al. Mechanical versus manual chest compressions for cardiac arrest. Cochrane Database Syst Rev 2014;(2): CD007260.

44. Gates S, Quinn T, Deakin CD, et al. Mechanical chest compression for out of hospital cardiac arrest: systematic review and meta-analysis. Resuscitation 2015;94:91–7.

45. Youngquist ST, Ockerse P, Hartsell S, et al. Mechanical chest compression devices are associated with poor neurological survival in a statewide registry: a propensity score analysis. Resuscitation 2016;106: 102–7.

46. Dobson R. How the power of touch reduces pain and even fights disease. Independent. 2006. Available at: http://www.independent.co.uk/life-style/health-and-families/health-news/how-the-power-of-touch-reduces-pain-and-even-fights-disease-419462.html. Accessed December 31, 2017.

Double Sequential Defibrillation

Erica M. Simon, DO, MHA[a], Kaori Tanaka, DO, MSPH[b],*

KEYWORDS

- Double sequential defibrillation • Defibrillation • Refractory ventricular fibrillation • Vector theory
- Threshold theory

KEY POINTS

- Refractory ventricular fibrillation is rare, occurring in 0.5 to 0.6 per 100,000 individuals.
- The mortality associated with refractory VF ranges from 85% to 97%.
- Current studies have demonstrated no statistically significant benefit of DSED, as compared with standard therapy, in terms of survival to hospital discharge and neurologic outcomes.

INTRODUCTION

Each year more than 300,000 out-of-hospital cardiac arrests (OHCA) occur in the United States.[1] In the setting of ventricular fibrillation (VF), the most frequently encountered tachyarrhythmia following spontaneous cardiac arrest, early defibrillation is paramount.[2,3] Today, communities equipped with mechanisms to ensure early defibrillation report mortality secondary to OHCA as 15% to 40%.[4–7] Although there is a clear benefit to the delivery of electricity during VF, the treatment of patients experiencing VF refractory to defibrillation remains a clinical concern.

REFRACTORY VENTRICULAR FIBRILLATION

Although there is no universal definition of refractory VF, it is generally considered to exist following three to five unsuccessful defibrillation attempts during adequate cardiopulmonary resuscitation.[8–11] Refractory VF is rare, with an estimated incidence of 0.5 to 0.6 episodes per 100,000 persons.[12] Individuals who experience refractory VF frequently have underlying structural heart disease and renal disease.[13–15] Additional risk factors for the development of refractory VF include advanced age, male sex, and reduced left ventricular ejection fraction.[13,14] Although interventions in the field may be limited, important precipitants for consideration include hypokalemia and hypomagnesemia.[14,16] Current studies estimate the mortality of refractory VF as 85% to 97%.[17,18] Although amiodarone and lidocaine represent the standard of care for the management of shock-refractory VF,[19] emergency medical services literature has placed an increasing focus on the potential role of prehospital double sequential defibrillation (DSED).

DOUBLE SEQUENTIAL DEFIBRILLATION

In the mid-1980s, electrophysiologists began the work of assessing methods of defibrillator shock delivery in canines.[20–22] Although research findings were variable among study groups, several investigators observed sequential shocks as reducing the total energy required to achieve successful defibrillation (laying the groundwork for the threshold theory: the first defibrillation lowers

Disclosure: The authors have nothing to disclose.
[a] Department of Emergency Medicine, San Antonio Uniformed Services Health Education Consortium, 3551 Roger Brooke Drive, Fort Sam Houston, TX 78234, USA; [b] Department of Emergency Medicine, University of Texas Health San Antonio, 7703 Floyd Curl Drive, MC 7736, San Antonio, TX 78229, USA
* Corresponding author.
E-mail address: tanakak@uthscsa.edu

Cardiol Clin 36 (2018) 387–393
https://doi.org/10.1016/j.ccl.2018.03.006

the threshold of success for the second defibrillation), and that the application of an additional electrode (a second vector), as increasing the likelihood of successful rhythm conversion (vector theory).[20,21] As applied to human models, proponents of the threshold and vector theories hypothesize that multiple shocks achieve a greater intracardiac current flow in the myocardium, thereby terminating VF, and that the application of an additional vector increases myocyte response, because cardiac fibers display directional sensitivity to electrical fields.[22–24] Today these mechanisms of action continue to be debated as some attribute the success of DSED to increased energy delivery (appropriate weight-based therapy).[25]

RESEARCH IN HUMAN SUBJECTS

In 1994, Hoch and colleagues[25] published the first human data regarding DSED.[25] In a randomized, controlled trial, the investigator and his colleagues demonstrated the safety and efficacy of sequential pulse shocks in the termination of refractory VF in five patients undergoing cardiac ablation. Since this time, DSED studies that require mention include those performed by Emmerson and colleagues,[26] Ross and colleagues,[29] Cabanas and colleagues,[11] Cortez and colleagues,[10] and Merlin and colleagues.[9] **Table 1** offers a summary of DSED literature.

In 2017, Emmerson and colleagues[26] published a retrospective observational analysis of patients who received DSED, performed by advanced paramedics of the London Ambulance Service. Of the 45 individuals experiencing refractory VF (42 males), return of spontaneous circulation (ROSC) was obtained in 17 following 2.5 ± 1.9 DSEDs (10 sustained ROSC until hospital arrival, DSED was performed following 10.2 ± 5.2 standard shocks, three survived to hospital discharge).[26] As compared with individuals receiving standard therapy (>6 standard shocks without DSED), no statistically significant differences in outcomes were observed (n = 175; mean age, 62.5 ± 16.5; 144 males; mean 10.4 ± 3.7 standard shocks; 11 survived to hospital discharge).[26] Mean time from dispatch to first defibrillation was $11:32 \pm 5:37$ for the DSED group and $12:22 \pm 4:50$ for the standard therapy group.[26]

Ross and colleagues,[29] in their performance of a retrospective cohort analysis, compared the neurologic outcomes of patients with presumed refractory or recurrent VF, treated in the prehospital setting with DSED (n = 50), with those who received standard therapy (single shocks;

n = 229). The authors' study revealed no statistically significant difference in cerebral performance categories (CPC) at hospital discharge. A total of 6% in the DSED group and 11.4% in the standard therapy group had CPC 1 or 2 at discharge (P = .317; odds ratio [OR], 0.50; 95% confidence interval [CI], 0.15–1.72).[29] Secondary outcomes of ROSC by EMS 28% versus 37.6% (P = .255; OR, 0.65; 95% CI, 0.33–1.27), survival to hospital admission 32% versus 35.4% (P = .744; OR, 0.86; 95% CI, 0.45–1.65), and survival to hospital discharge 8% versus 14.4% (P = .356; OR, 0.52; 95% CI, 0.17–1.53) also lacked statistical significance.[29] Subgroup analysis of patients with refractory VF (n = 26; defined as persisting in VF throughout the resuscitation) again noted no statistically significant difference in primary and secondary outcomes as compared with individuals having received standard therapy.[29]

Cabanas and colleagues,[11] reporting the first case series of DSED used in OHCA, identified a 70% termination of refractory VF following DSED in the prehospital setting (n = 10). Median age was 76.5 years (interquartile range [IQR], 65–82; median resuscitation time was 51 minutes (IQR, 45–62). However, ROSC was achieved in only three individuals, and none survived to hospital discharge.

In contrast to these studies, Cortez and colleagues[10] and Merlin and colleagues[9] offer evidence to suggest the potential for improved outcomes following DSED. Using data from the Columbus Division of Fire, Cortez and his colleagues conducted a retrospective review of patients who had received DSED in the prehospital setting from August 2010 to June 2014.[10] Of the 12 individuals included in the study, ROSC was achieved in three, and all three survived to hospital discharge (two with a CPC of 1, and one with a CPC of 3. Median prehospital resuscitation time was 31.5 minutes (IQR, 24–37.5), median time to DSED was 27 minutes (IQR, 22–33), median single defibrillation attempts were five (IQR, 5–6); and median dual defibrillation attempts were two (IQR, 1–2).[10]

In 2015, Merlin and colleagues[9] published a retrospective case series of patients receiving DSED for presumed refractory VF. Of the seven individuals included in the series, mean age was 62.9 (range, 45–78), mean resuscitation time was 34.3 minutes before first DSED (range, 10–48), mean number of single shocks was 5.4 before DSED (range, 3–9), a mean of two DSED shocks was delivered, VF was converted in five cases, and three individuals survived to hospital discharge with minimal neurologic impairment (CPC 1 or 2).[9]

Table 1
Summary of DSED literature

Authors	Study Design	Sample Characteristics	Pad Placement	DSD Attempts	ROSC	Survival to Hospital Discharge/CPC Score	Notes
Emmerson et al,[26] 2017	Retrospective observational analysis of patients who received DSED (July 2015–December 2016). Patients having received standard therapy (single shock) during the specified time frame offered as a comparison. Location: London.	DSED: 42 males, 3 females. Mean age: 59.8 ± 13. Standard therapy: 144 males, 31 females. Mean age: 62.5 ± 16.5.	DSED: A-L, A-P Standard: A-L	Mean: 2.5 ± 1.9	DSED: 17 (10 sustained ROSC to hospital). Standard: 61 (34 sustained ROSC to hospital).	DSED: 2 patients/not reported. Standard: 11 patients/not reported.	London Ambulance Service's advanced paramedics performed DSED. Per protocol, patients receive 6 standard shocks before DSD is attempted.
Tawil et al,[27] 2017	Case report. Location: Lebanon.	54-y-old man.	Not specified.	3	In emergency department.	Patient survived to discharge/ "neurologically intact."	
Cortez et al,[10] 2016	Retrospective chart review of VF patients treated with DSED in the prehospital setting (August 2010–June 2014). Location: Ohio.	11 males, 1 female (patient age data incomplete).	A-L, A-P	Mean: 1.75	3	3 patients/1, 1, and 3	Median prehospital resuscitation time: 31.5 min (IQR: 24–37.5). Mean standard shocks received: 4.6. Median time to DSD: 27 min (IQR: 22–33).
Johnston et al,[28] 2016	Case report. Location: Canada.	28-y-old woman.	A-L, A-P	1	Achieved on-scene.	Survived to discharge/2	Patient received 6 standard shocks before DSD.

(continued on next page)

Table 1
(continued)

Authors	Study Design	Sample Characteristics	Pad Placement	DSD Attempts	ROSC	Survival to Hospital Discharge/CPC Score	Notes
Merlin et al,[9] 2016	Retrospective case series of patients who received DSED (January 2015–April 2015). Location: New Jersey	4 males, 3 females. Mean age: 62. Mean weight: 84.2 kg.	A-L, A-P	Mean: 2	5 (4 survived to hospital)	3 Patients/mean: 3.4	Mean resuscitation time 34.4 min before DSD.
Ross et al,[29] 2016	Retrospective cohort analysis of prospectively collected quality assurance/quality improvement data (January 2013–December 2015). Patients having received standard therapy (single shocks) during the specified time frame offered as a comparison. Location: Texas.	DSED: 38 males, 12 females. Mean age: 59.4 y. Standard therapy: 168 males, 61 females. Mean age: 61.4.	DSD specified: A-P, A-S	Not reported.	DSED: 14. Standard: 86. Subgroup analysis: Refractory VF: 10.	DSED: 4/3 patients with CPC 1 or 2. Standard therapy: 33/26 patients with CPC 1 or 2. Refractory VF: 6/2 with CPC 1 or 2.	Study differentiated refractory and recurrent VF. Refractory VF defined as remaining in VF throughout the duration of the resuscitative effort.
Lybeck et al,[30] 2015	Case report. Location: Missouri.	40-y-old man.	A-L, A-P	1	In emergency department.	1/1	Patient received 7 standard shocks before DSD.

Cabanas et al,[11] 2015	Retrospective case series of adult patients with refractory VF (January 2008–December 2010). Location: North Carolina.	9 males, 1 female. Median age: 76.5 (IQR: 65–82).	A-L, A-P	Median: 2 (IQR 1–3)	3	0	Median resuscitation time: 51 min (IQR: 45–62). Median standard shocks: 6.5 (IQR: 6–11).
Leacock et al,[31,32] 2014	Case report. Location: St. Louis, Missouri.	51-y-old man. BMI: 39.8 kg/m²	A-L, A-P	1	In emergency department.	1/ "no neurologic impairment."	
Hoch et al,[25] 1994	Retrospective review of records: patients undergoing electrophysiologic studies (1990–1992). Location: Connecticut.	5 Males. Mean BMI: 34.9 kg/m² Mean left ventricular ejection fraction: 32	A-P, A-S	1	5	Not reported.	Shocks before DSED: 7–20. DSED shocks delivered 0.5–4.5 s apart.

Note: Gray: DSED performed in the prehospital setting.
Abbreviations: A-L, anterior-lateral; A-P, anterior-posterior; A-S, apex-sternum; BMI, body mass index; CPC, cerebral performance categories; DSD, double sequential defibrillation; IQR, interquartile range; ROSC, return of spontaneous circulation.

SUMMARY

To date, the two largest retrospective studies of DSED, both using data from the prehospital setting, have failed to demonstrate statistically significant improvements in patient survival and neurologic outcomes following the use of this defibrillation technique. At this point in time, the potential impact of DSED is unknown. Difficulty also exists when one considers confounding introduced by pharmacotherapy (eg, milligrams of epinephrine delivered). Encouragingly, a prospective study is on the horizon: a randomized, clinical trial, to be conducted by emergency medical services agencies, will soon be underway to assess patient outcomes following standard therapy, resuscitation involving DSED, and resuscitation involving vector change defibrillation.[31] It is hoped that this study may provide additional evidence to support or reject the practice of DSED.

REFERENCES

1. Keller S, Halperin H. Cardiac arrest: the changing incidence of ventricular fibrillation. Curr Treat Options Cardiovasc Med 2015;19(7):392.
2. Daya M, Schmicker R, Zive D. Out-of-hospital cardiac arrest survival improving over time: results from the Resuscitation Outcomes Consortium (ROC). Resuscitation 2015;91:108–15.
3. Chan P, Krumholz H, Nichol G, et al. Delayed time to defibrillation after in-hospital cardiac arrest. N Engl J Med 2008;358:9–17.
4. Stults K, Brown D, Schug V, et al. Prehospital defibrillation performed by emergency medical technicians in rural communities. N Engl J Med 1984;310:219–23.
5. Eisenberg M, Copass M, Hallstrom A, et al. Treatment of out-of-hospital cardiac arrests with rapid defibrillation by emergency medical technicians. N Engl J Med 1980;302:1379–83.
6. Valenzuela T, Spaite D, Meisline H, et al. Emergency vehicle intervals versus collapse-to-CPR and collapse-to-defibrillation intervals: monitoring emergency medical services system performance in sudden cardiac arrest. Ann Emerg Med 1993;22:1678–83.
7. Bunch T, White R, Gersch B, et al. Long-term outcomes of out-of-hospital cardiac arrest after successful early defibrillation. N Engl J Med 2003;348:2626–33.
8. Sarkozy A, Dorian P. Strategies for reversing shock-resistant ventricular fibrillation. Curr Opin Crit Care 2003;9:189–93.
9. Merlin M, Tagore A, Bauter R, et al. A case series of double sequential defibrillation. Prehosp Emerg Care 2016;20:550–3.
10. Cortez E, Krebs W, Davis J, et al. Use of double sequential external defibrillation for refractory ventricular fibrillation during out-of-hospital cardiac arrest. Resuscitation 2016;108:82–6.
11. Cabanas J, Myers J, Williams J, et al. Double sequential external defibrillation in out-of-hospital refractory ventricular fibrillation: a report of ten cases. Prehosp Emerg Care 2015;19:126–30.
12. Sakai T, Iwami T, Tasaki O, et al. Incidence and outcomes of out-of-hospital cardiac arrest with shock-resistant ventricular fibrillation: data from a large population-based cohort. Resuscitation 2010;81(8):956–61.
13. Villacastin J, Almendral J, Arenal A, et al. Incidence and clinical significance of multiple consecutive, appropriate, high-energy discharges in patients with implanted cardioverter-defibrillators. Circulation 1996;93(4):753–62.
14. Eifling M, Razavi M, Massumi A. The evaluation and management of electrical storm. Tex Heart Inst J 2011;38(2):111–21.
15. Gatzoulis K, Andrikopoulos G, Apostolopoulos T, et al. Electrical storm is an independent predictor of adverse long-term outcome in the era for implantable defibrillator therapy. Europace 2005;7(2):184–92.
16. European Heart Rhythm Association, Heart Rhythm Society, Zipes D, Camm A, Borggrefe M, et al. ACC/AHA/ESC 2006 guidelines for management of patients with ventricular arrhythmias and the prevention of sudden cardiac death: a report of the American College of Cardiology/American Heart Association Task Force and the European Society of Cardiology Committee for Practice Guidelines. J Am Coll Cardiol 2006;48(5):e247–346.
17. Windecker S. Percutaneous left ventricular assist devices for treatment of cardiogenic shock. Curr Opin Crit Care 2007;13(5):521–7.
18. Herlitz J, Bang A, Holmberg M, et al. Rhythm changes during resuscitation from ventricular fibrillation in relation to delay until defibrillation, number of shocks delivered and survival. Resuscitation 1997;34(1):17–22.
19. Kudenchuk P, Brown S, Daya M, et al. Resuscitation Outcomes Consortium – amiodarone, lidocaine, or placebo study (ROC-ALPS): rationale and methodology behind an out-of-hospital cardiac arrest antiarrhythmic drug trial. Am Heart J 2014;167(5):653–9.
20. Chang M, Inoue H, Kallok M, et al. Double and triple sequential shocks reduce ventricular defibrillation threshold in dogs with and without myocardial infarction. J Am Coll Cardiol 1986;8(6):1393–405.
21. Kerber R, Bourland J, Kallok M, et al. Transthoracic defibrillation using sequential and simultaneous dual shock pathways: experimental studies. Pacing Clin Electrophysiol 1990;13(2):201–17.
22. Frazier D, Krassowka W, Chen P, et al. Extracellular field required for excitation in three-dimensional

anisotropic canine myocardium. Circ Res 1988;63: 147–64.

23. Kerber R, Spencer K, Kallok M, et al. Overlapping sequential pulses: a new waveform for transthoracic defibrillation. Circulation 1994;89(5):2369–79.

24. Jones D, Klein G, Guiraudon G, et al. Biphasic versus sequential pulse defibrillation: a direct comparison in humans. Am Heart J 1993;125:405–9.

25. Hoch D, Batsford W, Greenberg S, et al. Double external shocks for refractory ventricular fibrillation. J Am Coll Cardiol 1994;23:1141–5.

26. Emmerson A, Whitbread M, Fothergill R. Double sequential defibrillation therapy for out-of-hospital arrests: the London experience. Resuscitation 2017;117:97–101.

27. Tawil C, Mrad S, Khishfe B. Double sequential defibrillation for refractory ventricular fibrillation. Am J Emerg Med 2017;35(12):1985.e3-4.

28. Johnston M, Cheskes S, Ross G, et al. Double sequential external defibrillation and survival from out-of-hospital cardiac arrest. Prehosp Emerg Care 2016;20(5):662–6.

29. Ross E, Redman T, Harper S, et al. Dual defibrillation in out-of-hospital cardiac arrest: a retrospective cohort analysis. Resuscitation 2016;106:14–7.

30. Lybeck A, Moy H, Tan D. Double sequential defibrillation for refractory ventricular fibrillation, a case report. Prehosp Emerg Care 2015;19(4):554–7.

31. Leacock B. Double simultaneous defibrillators for refractory ventricular fibrillation. J Emerg Med 2014; 46(4):472–4.

32. Sunnybrook Health Sciences Centre. Double sequential external defibrillation for refractory VF (DOSE-VF). Available at: https://clinicaltrials.gov/show/NCT03249948. Accessed December 13, 2017.

Management of Refractory Ventricular Fibrillation (Prehospital and Emergency Department)

Sean M. Bell, MD[a], David H. Lam, MD[a,b],
Kathleen Kearney, MD[a,b], Ravi S. Hira, MD[a,b,c],*

KEYWORDS

- Refractory ventricular fibrillation • Urgent coronary angiography • Out-of-hospital cardiac arrest
- Extracorporeal membrane oxygenation • Mechanical cardiopulmonary resuscitation

KEY POINTS

- Refractory ventricular fibrillation carries a high mortality rate, and often does not respond to conventional therapy.
- Most patients presenting with out-of-hospital cardiac arrest and refractory ventricular fibrillation have an acute thrombotic coronary artery lesion; urgent coronary angiography with revascularization is critical.
- Extracorporeal membrane oxygenation allows providers additional time to diagnose and treat potentially reversible causes of ventricular fibrillation-associated cardiac arrest.
- Novel multifaceted approaches for the management of refractory ventricular fibrillation have provided encouraging results.

 Video content accompanies this article at www.cardiology.theclinics.com.

INTRODUCTION

Ventricular fibrillation (VF) is a potentially fatal, life-threatening cardiac arrhythmia that can lead to loss of cardiac function and sudden cardiac death. VF is characterized on an electrocardiogram (ECG) as irregular and disorganized electrical activity without any discernible pattern. With an annual incidence of 12.1 per 100,000 people, VF remains the leading cause of sudden cardiac death and out-of-hospital cardiac arrest (OHCA).[1] Prompt treatment with resuscitation and defibrillation can be life saving and, therefore, recognition of VF by first responders and medical professionals is essential. However, an estimated 4% to 5% of OHCA is characterized by VF that does not respond to multiple attempts at defibrillation, a phenomenon known as refractory VF. The incidence of refractory VF is estimated at 0.5 to 0.6 per 100,000 people.[2]

Despite improvement in survival rates of patients experiencing OHCA, survival in the subset of patients with refractory VF remains poor.[2] Mortality rates among patients with refractory VF

Disclosure: R.S. Hira is a consultant for Abbott Vascular, Inc. S.M. Bell, D. H. Lam, and K. Kearney have nothing to disclose.
[a] Department of Medicine, University of Washington, 1959 Northeast Pacific Street, Seattle, WA 98195, USA;
[b] Division of Cardiology, University of Washington, 1959 Northeast Pacific Street, Seattle, WA 98195, USA;
[c] Department of Medicine, Division of Cardiology, Harborview Medical Center, 325 Ninth Avenue, Seattle, WA 98104, USA
* Corresponding author. 325 Ninth Avenue, Box 359748, Seattle, WA 98104.
E-mail address: hira@uw.edu

Cardiol Clin 36 (2018) 395–408
https://doi.org/10.1016/j.ccl.2018.03.007
0733-8651/18/© 2018 Elsevier Inc. All rights reserved.

range between 85% and 97%, and the proportion of patients with neurologically intact function at 1 month after refractory VF is estimated at only 5.6%.[2,3] By contrast, patients who present with OHCA and an initial shockable rhythm have a survival to hospital discharge rate of 33.0%, with survival with good neurologic function of 30.1% as reported in the Cardiac Arrest Registry to Enhance Survival (CARES) in 2015.[4] This finding highlights a need for early detection and improved intervention for patients who suffer from refractory VF.

Normal cardiac electrophysiology requires intricate, spontaneous, automatic, and synchronized signaling within the cardiomyocytes. Typically, the electric signal originates from pacemaker cells in the sinoatrial node in the right atrium. The signal then continues toward the atrioventricular node and, ultimately, through the ventricles producing synchronized muscular contraction. Under normal conditions, atrial and ventricular myocytes do not spontaneously depolarize. If, however, ventricular cardiomyocytes have endured damage in some form, they can become prone to electrical hyperexcitability and depolarization without a signal from the sinoatrial node. This scenario is most applicable to patients who experience acute myocardial injury, usually from ischemic events. Without synchrony, there is a loss of coordinated contraction and reduced cardiac output. This situation, in turn, leads to a vicious cycle of continued ischemic damage and further deterioration of the electrophysiologic integrity of the myocardium. By ECG, this cycle manifests as increased fibrillation cycle length of the ventricles (ie, VF) and the usual P, QRS, and T wave morphologies are replaced with an erratic rhythm. This pattern results in mechanical dyssynchrony without adequate ventricular ejection and stroke volume. Without intervention, the VF rhythm eventually progresses to asystole and death.

In this review, we summarize therapeutic interventions and guidelines to provide guidance to clinicians managing patients with OHCA and refractory VF, both in the prehospital and emergency department (ED) setting. The approach to VF focuses on initiation of aggressive resuscitation and supportive care, which includes advanced cardiac life support (ACLS), restoration of normal electrical activity by defibrillation and/or medical therapy, followed by appropriate postresuscitation care after return of spontaneous circulation (ROSC). This process includes hemodynamic stabilization, prompt investigation for the underlying etiology of VF, and targeted temperature management (TTM) when indicated. Investigation of the underlying etiology is done with a history and physical examination, laboratory results, imaging, and ancillary investigation, which may include coronary angiography. In patients with refractory VF who do not have ROSC, however, there is currently no accepted consensus on management after failed defibrillation and resuscitation attempts. Here, we discuss a strategy of limited duration of resuscitative efforts in the field followed by prompt transfer to a facility capable of immediately initiating use of venoarterial extracorporeal membrane oxygenation (ECMO) in these patients followed by cardiac catheterization and revascularization.

CURRENT GUIDELINES

Current management guidelines for VF emphasize the importance of early, high-quality cardiopulmonary resuscitation (CPR) at a rate of 100 to 120 compressions per minute.[5] Ventilatory support is provided at a rate of 2 breaths for every 30 compressions or 1 breath every 6 seconds if an advanced airway is in place. After the initiation of CPR, use of an automated external defibrillator (AED) should be implemented rapidly with the defibrillation pads placed and cardiac rhythm assessment performed. If this process identifies a shockable rhythm, the shock should be delivered as soon as possible. If a biphasic AED is in use, the initial shock energy delivered is based on the manufacturer's recommendation. If the manufacturer's recommendation is unknown, then the highest energy level available is recommended (typically 200 J). For a monophasic AED, the recommended shock energy is 360 J. CPR is then resumed immediately for 2 minutes, during which time vascular access should be attained. CPR is continued in 2-minute intervals, with rhythm checks performed every 2 minutes. If ROSC is achieved, the patient is then immediately transitioned to post–cardiac arrest care. If ROSC is not achieved, and the rhythm check continues to show VF, a shock should be delivered with immediate resumption of CPR. After the second defibrillation attempt, 1 mg of epinephrine either intravenous or intraosseous every 3 to 5 minutes is recommended. After the third defibrillation attempt, an initial amiodarone load of 300 mg administered intravenously or intraosseously is recommended, followed by doses of 150 mg. If the patient remains in VF despite 3 defibrillation attempts and optimal medical therapy, we would define this as refractory VF with a significant decrease in anticipated survival.[6]

CARDIOPULMONARY RESUSCITATION

Early recognition and intervention of patients with OHCA is critical for patient survival. In a nationwide study in Denmark of 2855 patients who were 30-day survivors after OHCA, bystander resuscitation and defibrillation were associated with significantly lower rates of brain damage and death from any cause compared with those who did not receive bystander resuscitation or defibrillation.[7] Several factors influence the rate of bystander CPR, including race, ethnicity, socioeconomic status, and country.[8–10] Significant efforts have been made to increase the rates of bystander CPR including school-based CPR training, mandating CPR as a prerequisite to other activities (ie, attaining a driver's license), and mobile phone apps for self-directed CPR training.[11–14]

Although manual chest compressions remain the standard of care for patients with OHCA, maintaining high-quality manual chest compressions can be difficult.[15(p6)] Provider fatigue, patient access, and extended interruptions can lead to a decrease in the quality of manual CPR delivered.[16] Mechanical compression devices that are gas or electric powered pistons can be positioned over the sternum of a patient to deliver chest compressions at a set rate. Two large randomized controlled trials enrolling a combined 7060 patients comparing mechanical CPR with standard of care, found no difference in survival at 1 to 6 months.[17,18] A recent prospective observational study of 6537 patients found a decreased likelihood of survival to hospital discharge (adjusted odds ratio [OR], 0.40; 95% confidence interval [CI], 0.20–0.78; $P = .005$), ROSC (adjusted OR, 0.71; 95% CI, 0.53–0.94; $P = .018$), and hospital admission (adjusted OR, 0.57; 95% CI, 0.40–0.80; $P = .001$) with mechanical CPR compared with those receiving manual CPR.[19] Notably, only 14% of these patients (918 of 6537) received mechanical CPR. The routine use of mechanical CPR devices is not currently recommended; however, guidelines suggest their use in situations in which manual CPR may be difficult, such as in a moving ambulance or angiography suite (Video 1).[15(p6)] The LUCAS device (Physio-Control Inc., Redmond, WA), for example, is able to provide mechanical CPR with a radiolucent back plate enabling coronary angiography and intervention (**Fig. 1**).

DEFIBRILLATION

Defibrillation is a potentially life-saving intervention and remains definitive therapy for patients with VF. With the advent of AEDs, first responders and even bystanders can intervene with relative ease before EMS arrival. Indeed, improved survival rates among patients experiencing OHCA may largely be attributed to improvement in basic

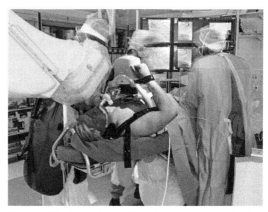

Fig. 1. Mechanical cardiopulmonary resuscitation device.

life support and ACLS implementation in conjunction with widespread distribution of AEDs. Defibrillators using biphasic waveforms are associated with high rates of atrial and ventricular arrhythmia termination, and are the preferred modality of defibrillation by the American Heart Association (AHA; class IIa, level of evidence [LOE] B-R).[5] Biphasic waveform AEDs are further subdivided in to biphasic truncated exponential defibrillators, rectilinear biphasic defibrillators, and pulsed biphasic waveforms. Currently, there is no conclusive evidence to support the use of one form of biphasic AED as compared with another for the termination of VF. In light of this finding, current recommendations are to administer the manufacturer's recommended energy dose for the first shock.[5]

Alternatives to standard defibrillation protocols for patients with refractory VF have recently been reported in the literature,[20,21] including double sequential defibrillation (DSD) and stacked sequential defibrillation. DSD uses a second set of defibrillation pads for a patient with refractory VF and ongoing resuscitation. Typically, 1 set of pads is placed in the anteroposterior orientation, with the second set placed in an anterolateral orientation. Both defibrillators are set at their highest energy delivery level, and the shock is delivered simultaneously. The mechanism by which DSD promotes ROSC in patients with refractory VF as compared with standard single shock protocols is unclear, although it is speculated to be related to increased defibrillation vectors, and more energy delivered across the myocardium with each defibrillation attempt. Currently, no case-control studies exist to guide the use of DSD in patients with refractory VF; however, given the noninvasive nature of DSD and the ease of implementation en route to the hospital, the use of DSD remains an attractive option for EMS personnel. One randomized controlled trial compared the standard of care single shock protocol and 2 minutes of CPR with a 3-sequential shock protocol and 1 minute of CPR. There were no differences in survival at 1 year between the protocols.[22] Therefore, single shock therapy remains the AHA recommended option for defibrillation (class IIa; LOE B-NR).[5]

Although guidelines vary by institution, typically EMS responders perform at least 3 defibrillation attempts before initiating hospital transportation. Importantly, rates of survival are inversely proportional to the number of shocks administered to achieve ROSC.[6] Furthermore, the success of defibrillation decreases by as much as 7% for each minute of untreated VF or ventricular tachycardia (VT). Thus, should the patient remain in VF after 3 defibrillation attempts, further intervention beyond the standard ACLS protocol will likely be needed. In patients with refractory VF, continuing resuscitative efforts in the field are likely to be futile, and an aggressive strategy of immediate transport with mechanical CPR (class IIb; LOE B), initiation of hemodynamic support with venoarterial ECMO (class IIb; LOE C-LD), and immediate coronary angiography and percutaneous coronary intervention (PCI) would be recommended (class IIa; LOE-B).

MEDICAL THERAPY
Antiarrhythmic Medications

Antiarrhythmic medications are commonly used in patients with OHCA (**Table 1**). Patients with refractory VF are likely to have underlying coronary vessel occlusion and, therefore, are unlikely to convert to an organized perfusing rhythm with the use of pharmacologic therapy alone.[5] Previous studies had demonstrated that intravenous administration of amiodarone therapy after at least 3 failed defibrillation attempts in patients with refractory VF was associated with improved survival to hospital admission rates as compared with placebo and lidocaine.[23] A recent randomized, double-blinded trial compared the use of lidocaine and amiodarone in patients with nontraumatic OHCA with an initial rhythm of VF or pulseless VT (pVT), and found no improvement in neurologic outcomes or survival rates as compared with placebo.[24] Current ACLS guidelines recommend consideration of amiodarone therapy in patients with VF/pVT who are unresponsive to CPR, defibrillation, and vasopressor therapy, administered in an initial 300 mg bolus followed 150 mg doses (class IIb; LOE B-R).[5] Routine lidocaine use is not recommended but may be considered after ROSC from VT/VF arrest.

Vasoactive Agents

Hypotension is common in patients presenting with OHCA and should be treated to maintain adequate perfusion pressure. Epinephrine provides vasopressor support by stimulating alpha-adrenergic receptors in the vasculature.[25] Stimulation of alpha-adrenergic receptors leads to vasoconstriction and increase in systemic pressure. Epinephrine is administered in 1-mg doses intravenously or intraosseously every 3 to 5 minutes during resuscitation (class IIb; LOE B-R). The use of epinephrine has long been a staple of the ACLS protocol. These recommendations are largely based on animal studies[26,27] because the use of epinephrine in cardiac arrest has not been shown conclusively in any human clinical trials.[28] Although evidence remains sparse, 1 randomized placebo controlled trial found a significantly improved likelihood of achieving ROSC in patients presenting with OHCA who received epinephrine as compared with placebo (23.5% vs 8.4%; OR, 3.4; 95% CI, 0.7–6.3).[29] No statistically significant difference in survival to hospital discharge was observed between the 2 treatment arms, although the study was stopped early because it was underpowered to assess these outcomes.

There have been numerous trials comparing the use of high-dose epinephrine (0.1–0.2 mg/kg) with standard dose epinephrine.[30–32] Outcome measures in these trials included survival to hospital admission, survival to hospital discharge, and survival to hospital discharge with good neurologic recovery. There did not seem to be any benefit for the use of high-dose epinephrine as compared with standard dose epinephrine among these outcomes. Consequently, the AHA recommends against the use of high-dose epinephrine for the routine use in cardiac arrest patients.[5] In a recent 2×2 porcine model of ischemic refractory VF, Bartos and colleagues[33] randomized animals to the use of epinephrine or placebo during ACLS and then again randomized to ECMO or no ECMO at the time of reinitiation of coronary flow. The primary study endpoint was survival at 4 hours. In pigs receiving repeated epinephrine boluses compared with placebo, although there was an increase in systemic blood pressure and coronary perfusion pressure, there was no difference in survival (47% vs 69%; $P = .47$). There was, however, a significant increase in survival of pigs receiving ECMO as compared with those that did not (82% vs 31%; $P = .003$). This study suggests that the role of epinephrine in ischemic refractory VF is limited because it did not seem appear to offer any advantage in survival or ROSC as compared with placebo. Standard dose

Table 1
Summary of commonly administered medications during ventricular fibrillation cardiac arrest

Trial Name, Year	No. of Patients	Medication	Dosing	Frequency	Indication	AHA Guidelines (2015)
ALIVE,[60] 2002 ARREST,[23] 1999	347 504	Amiodarone	300 mg or 5 mg/kg with a repeat dose of 150 mg IV as indicated	Maximum recommended total daily dose is 2.2 g	VF or pulseless VT unresponsive to defibrillation ×3 cycles, CPR, and epinephrine	First-line therapy antiarrhythmic
ALIVE, 2002 Kudenchuk et al,[24] 2016	347 3026	Lidocaine	1–1.5 mg/kg IV, then 0.5–0.75 mg/kg	Every 5–10 min with a maximum of 3 doses or total of 3 mg/kg	VF or pulseless VT unresponsive to defibrillation ×3 cycles, CPR, and epinephrine	Second-line therapy, if no access to amiodarone
Tzivoni et al,[61] 1988	12	Magnesium	2 g IV push	Maintenance infusion after bolus	VF or pulseless VT arrest owing to drug-induced prolonged QT interval associated with torsades de pointes	Only to be used if managing torsades de pointes

Abbreviations: AHA, American Heart Association; CPR, cardiopulmonary resuscitation; IV, intravenous; VF, ventricular fibrillation; VT, ventricular tachycardia.

epinephrine has also been compared with the use of vasopressin in 1 randomized clinical trial of 336 patient presenting with cardiac arrest.[34] This trial showed no benefit with use of vasopressin as compared with epinephrine for survival to hospital discharge or ROSC. Vasopressin has since been removed from the ACLS Adult Cardiac Arrest Algorithm.

Recently, esmolol has been studied as an adjuvant therapy in patients who have refractory VF. Continued administration of epinephrine stimulates not only alpha receptors leading to vasoconstriction and increased myocardial perfusion, but also beta 1 and 2 receptors, which increases myocardial oxygen demand, and reduced subendocardial perfusion, which may worsen ischemic injury and overall myocardial function.[5,26,35] A systematic review of the use of beta-blockade therapy in animal models as well as 2 human prospective studies suggests that it may be useful during cardiac arrest.[36] In a small retrospective study of patients with VF or pVT, among patients who received esmolol after at least 3 defibrillation attempts, 300 mg of amiodarone, and 3 mg of epinephrine, compared with standard of care, there was an increase in the rate of ROSC (66.7% vs 31.6%, respectively) as well as survival benefit (50% vs 15.8%, respectively) in patients who received esmolol, although these findings were not statistically significant given the limited sample size (esmolol group, n = 6; no esmolol group, n = 19).[37] Notably, 1 patient experienced a bradycardic pulseless electrical activity arrest. Further study is required to elucidate the role of esmolol in patients with refractory VF. There are no current guidelines for the routine use of esmolol in patients with refractory VF.

Neuroprotective Agents

In experimental animal models of cardiac arrest, sodium nitrite limited acute cardiac dysfunction, neurologic impairment, and death in survivors.[38–40] Cardioprotective and neuroprotective effects were observed when blood levels of sodium nitrite reached 12 μmol/L and 19 μmol/L, respectively.[38,40] A recent pilot study evaluating the hemodynamic effects of sodium nitrite therapy in patients with OHCA showed no significant hemodynamic changes as compared with placebo, suggesting that sodium nitrite can be safely administered in this patient population.[41] A phase I open-label trial (NCT02987088) evaluating the plasma level of sodium nitrite in patients with OHCA who receive 25 mg intravenous of sodium nitrite has recently completed enrollment. The second phase will be a placebo-control, randomized trial of the sodium nitrite delivered during resuscitation to determine safety and efficacy.

TARGETED TEMPERATURE MANAGEMENT

One of the most common adverse outcomes after cardiac arrest is neurologic injury.[42] TTM has been shown to improve neurologic function and survival after cardiac arrest.[43,44] More recently, Nielsen and colleagues[45] conducted a large multicenter randomized trial comparing outcomes for TTM at 33°C versus 36°C in 939 patients who had been resuscitated after OHCA of suspected cardiac etiology. There was no statistically significant difference in all-cause mortality in patients managed with TTM of 33°C as compared with 36°C (hazard ratio, 1.06; 95% CI, 0.89–1.28; $P = .51$). In addition, there was no difference in neurologic function or death assessed at 180 days. These results suggested that TTM directed to 33°C did not improve all-cause mortality or neurologic outcomes when compared with 36°C. Several methods to initiate and maintain TTM are available (**Table 2**) and are beyond the scope of this review. However, it is important to point out that the optimal time from initiation of treatment to achievement of targeted temperature as well as the total duration of therapy remains uncertain.

Currently, the AHA recommends selecting and maintaining a constant temperature between 32°C and 36°C as a class I (LOE B-R) indication for patients after cardiac arrest that have achieved ROSC.[46] Furthermore, the AHA recommends maintaining TTM for at least 24 hours after achievement of targeted temperature (class IIa; LOE C-EO). This intervention can be instituted in either the prehospital and ED settings. Notably, these same guidelines recommend against cooling with rapid infusion of intravenous fluids. These recommendations are based on 5 randomized control trials showing no benefit with regard to survival or neurologic recovery, although 1 trial showed in an increase in pulmonary edema.[47] The optimal strategy of TTM in patients with refractory VF that have not achieved ROSC is not known.

URGENT CORONARY ANGIOGRAPHY

In the context of OHCA with suspected cardiac etiology, it is important to identify the inciting pathology leading to cardiac arrest. The most common reason for OHCA is coronary artery disease (CAD), with 50% to 60% of patients found to have a culprit lesion identified on coronary angiography.[48,49] Thus, urgent coronary angiography and revascularization, if needed, is critical. In

Table 2
Summary of targeted temperature management studies

Study, Year	No. of Patients	Intervention Arms	Inclusion Criteria	Primary Outcomes and Results	Secondary Outcomes and Results
HACA,[44] 2002	275	32° to 34°C vs standard ICU care	Either out or in-hospital VF or VT Comatose Witnessed arrest Age 18–75 y	Favorable neurologic outcome within 6 mo: 55% vs 39% (RR, 1.40; 95% CI, 1.08–1.81; P<.009; NNT, 6)	Overall mortality at 6 mo: 41% vs 55% (RR, 0.74; 95% CI, 0.58–0.95; P<.02; NNT, 7) Rate of complications during the first 7 d after cardiac arrest (bleeding, pneumonia, sepsis, pancreatitis, renal failure, pulmonary edema, seizures, arrhythmias, and pressure sores): 73% vs 70% (P<.70)
Bernard et al,[43] 2002	77	33°C vs standard ICU care	Out of hospital VF Comatose Age ≥18 for men Age ≥50 for women	Survival to hospital discharge with good neurologic function: 49% vs 26% (P = .046), adjusted OR, 5.25 (95% CI, 1.47–18.76; P = .011)	Hemodynamic, biochemical and hematologic complications: no statistically significant differences
Laurent et al,[62] 2005	42	32° to 33°C vs 37°C	Out of hospital VF or asystole Comatose Age 18–75 y	Survival with a follow-up time of 6 mo: • HF + HT: 32% • HF: 45% • Control: 21% (P = .018) (95% CI, 1.1–16.6)	Effect of HF on death by intractable shock (P = .0009): • HF + HT: 14% (RR, 0.29; 95% CI, 0.09–0.91) • HF: 10% (RR, 0.21;95% CI, 0.05–0.85) • Control: 42%

(continued on next page)

Table 2
(continued)

Study, Year	No. of Patients	Intervention Arms	Inclusion Criteria	Primary Outcomes and Results	Secondary Outcomes and Results
TTM,[45] 2013	939	33° vs 36°C	Out of hospital Age ≥18 Comatose All rhythms ROSC of ≥20 min	All-cause mortality: 50% vs 48% of the patients in the 36°C group (225 of 466 patients) (HR, 1.06; 95% CI, 0.89–1.28; P = .51)	Survival to hospital discharge with good neurologic function: 54% vs 52% (HR, 1.02; 95% CI, 0.88–1.16; P = .78) Death at 180 d: 48% vs 47% (HR, 1.01; 95% CI, 0.87–1.15; P = .92)
Bray et al,[63] 2017	76	33° vs 36°C	Out of hospital VF	Percentage at TT: 87% vs 50% (P<.001)	Survival overall: 71% vs 55% (P = .31) Survival to hospital discharge with good neurologic function: 71% vs 56% (P = .22) Discharge home: 82% vs 73% (P = .08)
Prehospital hypothermia					
Kim et al,[47] 2007	125	2L 4°C NS vs standard of care (including therapeutic hypothermia in ICU)	Out of hospital All rhythms ROSC Age ≥18 y IV access	Temperature difference: 34.7°C ± 1.2°C vs 35.7°C ± 1.2°C (P<.0001)	Survival overall: 32% vs 29% Note: Trend toward better outcomes in patients with VF (66% vs 45% discharged alive)
Kämäräinen et al,[64] 2009	43	33°C vs standard of care	Out of hospital All rhythms ROSC >9 min Age ≥18 y IV access	Nasopharyngeal temperature at time of arrival to ED: 34.1°C ± 0.9°C vs 35.2°C ± 0.8°C (P<.001)	Survival to hospital discharge with good neurologic function: no statistical difference (42% vs 44%) despite faster cooling times achieved

Abbreviations: CI, confidence interval; HF, heart failure; HR, hazard ratio; HT, hypothermia; ICU, intensive care unit; IV, intravenous; NNT, number needed to treat; NS, normal saline; ROSC, return of spontaneous circulation; RR, relative risk; TT, target temperature; VF, ventricular fibrillation; VT, ventricular tachycardia.

resuscitated OHCA patients, evidence of a shockable rhythm such as VF or pVT, ST segment elevation on ECG, and a history of CAD were associated with urgent coronary angiography within 6 hours of presentation.[50] Once a culprit lesion is identified, myocardial reperfusion can be achieved with PCI if indicated.

Given the high rate of CAD, culprit lesions, and coronary occlusion in patients presenting with OHCA as well as the poor predictive value of ECGs in patients after resuscitation from cardiac arrest, some investigators also advocate for the routine use of coronary angiography and PCI in patients without ST segment elevation on ECG.[49,51,52] If a culprit lesion is present, intervention could salvage myocardium as well as prevent rearrest. The other advantage of taking these critically ill patients to the cardiac catheterization laboratory (CCL) is assessment of invasive hemodynamics via right heart catheterization and implementation of mechanical circulatory support through devices such as an intraaortic balloon pump therapy or temporary ventricular support devices such as the Impella (ABIOMED, Danvers, MA).

The majority of patients presenting with OHCA and refractory VF have an acute thrombotic lesion.[53] Therefore, earlier ascertainment of VF that is refractory followed by invasive attempts to treat the lesion may improve survival in these patients compared with continued noninvasive management in the field. This factor presents a challenge in determining the optimal duration of resuscitation to "stay and play" in the field and when to "pack and ship" a patient to a hospital where advanced therapies could be delivered. An important role of prehospital and ED providers is, therefore, rapid identification of patients who have refractory VF in the field for immediate transport to a facility where appropriate advanced therapy and protocols to care for these patients and address the underlying coronary occlusion are available, as well as prehospital activation of the CCL and advanced therapy processes. It is important to note that this destination may not be the nearest hospital or hospital with PCI capability, but centers of excellence with experience in caring for these patients.

EXTRACORPOREAL MEMBRANE OXYGENATION

ECMO is an emerging therapeutic intervention for patients with cardiac arrest, both outside and within hospitals, in patients who require complete hemodynamic support after initial attempts at stabilization have proved unsuccessful. ECMO involves cannulation of the arterial and venous systems, typically by way of the femoral vessels, and initiation of artificial oxygenation and circulation (**Fig. 2**). In patients with refractory VF, the use of ECMO may allow providers additional time to diagnose and treat potentially reversible causes of VF-associated cardiac arrest. When performed in patients with ongoing CPR, the terms ECMO-CPR or ECPR are used.

Given the resource-intensive nature of ECMO along with the high rate of mortality of patients who receive ECMO, early risk stratification is desirable. Lactate, bilirubin, and International Normalized Ratio have demonstrated predictive value in patients who undergo ECMO, because elevated levels of these markers are associated with higher rates of mortality.[54] In addition, a French guideline from 2009 suggests using end-tidal carbon dioxide levels of 10 mm Hg or greater as a guide to initiating ECMO, because values less than this are associated with poor neurologic prognosis.[55] In an effort to predict survival and judiciously use ECMO in patients with refractory VF, the Survival After Venoarterial ECMO (SAVE) score was

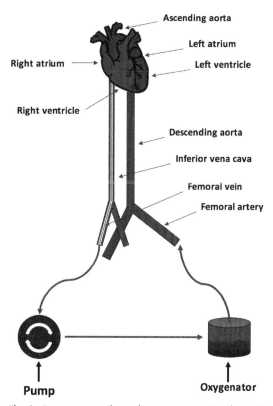

Fig. 2. Extracorporeal membrane oxygenation (ECMO) involves cannulation of the arterial and venous systems, and initiation of artificial oxygenation and circulation. (*Courtesy of* Anna Cummings Rork, MD, Seattle, WA.)

developed as a guide for clinicians. Formulated with data from an international cohort of 3846 patients admitted for OHCA, the SAVE score incorporates 12 separate risk factors used to calculate survival probability. The SAVE score has since been modified with new data demonstrating the usefulness of lactate for patients with refractory VF requiring ECMO.[56]

The AHA and International Liaison Committee on Resuscitation 2015 review guidelines recommend consideration of ECMO in patients presenting with cardiac arrest from presumed reversible etiology, including myocardial infarction, pulmonary embolism, and refractory VF (class IIb; LOE C-LE).[5]

NOVEL STRATEGIES FOR REFRACTORY VENTRICULAR FIBRILLATION ARREST

With growing data to suggest survival benefit with use of early invasive strategies, including early coronary angiography and ECMO, novel multifaceted strategies incorporating these therapies are becoming more prevalent.

The CHEER (mechanical CPR, Hypothermia, ECMO, and Early Reperfusion) trial incorporated mechanical CPR, TTM, ECMO, and early reperfusion in the management of patients with refractory cardiac arrest in both prehospital and hospital settings.[57] Included in this study were patients aged 18 to 65 years, presenting with cardiac arrest of suspected cardiac etiology who had initial rhythms of VF, and in whom chest compressions were initiated within 10 minutes of arrest in locations where mechanical CPR was available. Hypothermia was achieved with the rapid infusion of 2 L cold saline en route to the hospital, and patients were maintained at a core body temperature of 33°C for 24 hours. Patients with suspected coronary artery occlusion were taken urgently to the CCL. Primary outcome data included survival to hospital discharge with good neurologic outcomes measured with a Cerebral Performance Category (CPC) scores of 1 or 2. Of the patients presenting with OHCA, 73% suffered from acute coronary syndrome (n = 11). Five of these patients (45%) survived to hospital discharge with good neurologic outcomes (CPC of 1 or 2). Statistically significant variations between the survivors and nonsurvivors in this study included the difference in median time from cardiac event to initiation of ECMO (40 minutes vs 78 minutes, respectively; $P = .02$). Although further study is needed to evaluate the usefulness of this protocol, particularly the resource implications of ECMO and mechanical CPR, the CHEER trial suggests a multifaceted approach for patients with refractory cardiac arrest may lead to reduced morbidity and mortality in this population.

More recently, Yannopoulos and colleagues[53] evaluated the survival of patients presenting with VF-associated OHCA treated with mechanical CPR, early ECMO, and revascularization, as compared with historical controls who had received the standard of care. Patients included in this study were those with an initial presenting rhythm of VF/VT, aged 18 to 75, whose body habitus could accommodate a LUCAS-automated CPR device, who had received at least 3 defibrillation attempts, 300 mg intravenous or intraosseous amiodarone, and were located within an estimated transfer time from the scene to the CCL of less than 30 minutes. Excluded from this study were patients with cardiac arrest of noncardiac etiology, nursing home residents, the presence of a valid do not resuscitate or do not intubate order, contraindications to mechanical CPR, and those with terminal illness. Although TTM was not a specific therapeutic modality, all patients arriving for invasive intervention were hypothermic (average core temperature of 34°C) and subsequently maintained for 24 hours with the exception of patients who experienced bleeding complications. Patients undergoing early ECMO had dramatically improved functional survival rates with CPC scores of 1 or 2 compared with historical controls (43% vs 15.3%; OR, 4.0; 95% CI, 2.08–7.7; $P<.001$). Interestingly, patients who survived to discharge had a higher rate of CAD, suggesting that early identification and treatment of culprit lesions, when present, improves survival.

Although the initial results of novel multimodal approaches to refractory VF are encouraging, further study is required to define the population that would benefit from such an aggressive invasive approach. The Prague OHCA study[58] (NCT01511666), is an ongoing prospective randomized trial initiated in 2012 comparing a hyperinvasive approach to standard therapy in patients with witnessed OHCA of presumed cardiac origin. Patients randomized to the hyperinvasive arm receive mechanical CPR, intranasal evaporative cooling, initiation of venoarterial ECMO within 60 minutes from time of collapse, and early coronary angiography. Primary inclusion criteria include witnessed OHCA of presumed cardiac etiology, age between 18 and 65 years, a minimum of 5 minutes of ACLS performed by EMS without sustained ROSC, unconsciousness, and the availability of ECMO team and intensive care bed capacity at a nearby cardiac center. Primary exclusion criteria include OHCA of presumed noncardiac etiology, unwitnessed collapse, confirmed or suspected pregnancy, consciousness, ROSC attained within 5 minutes of ACLS, known CPC score of 3 or greater, the presence of a do not resuscitate order, suspected or confirmed stroke, severe chronic organ dysfunction, and suspected or confirmed acute or recent intracranial bleeding. The primary outcome assessed is the 6-month survival with good neurologic function (CPC score of 1–2). The Prague study is expected to complete enrollment of an anticipated 170 patients in 2018.

As mentioned, there is a fine balance between spending time providing high-quality resuscitation in the field and not delaying transport for advanced therapies such as ECMO and PCI in patients with refractory VF. There is a significant association between CPR duration and mortality with patients that receive CPR for 45 minutes of less before being placed on ECMO having improved survival to discharge compared with patients receiving more than 45 minutes of CPR. Survival decreased significantly after 60 minutes.[59] These data suggest that early initiation of ECMO in these patients is critical. One of the potential solutions for the dilemma of optimal timing for transport to a hospital is to bring ECMO to the patients and initiate ECMO in the field. A comparative study between prehospital and in-hospital ECMO for patients with refractory cardiac arrest is currently enrolling study participants (NCT02527031). Investigators aim to initiate ECMO in the field within 30 minutes of cardiac arrest. Results of this study are expected in 2019.

OUR APPROACH

Our center's approach to VF arrest is multifaceted. For patients who achieve ROSC in the field, guideline directed care including an immediate postresuscitation ECG is performed. If there is ST segment elevation, the CCL is emergently activated and immediate coronary angiography is performed. If there are no ST segment elevations, a TTM protocol is initiated on arrival to the ED and an expedited evaluation for the cause of arrest is performed. This evaluation includes a history and physical examination to look for trauma and bleeding, and laboratory analysis to evaluate for reversible metabolic and toxic derangements. A comprehensive computed tomography scan protocoled to rule out multiple causes of arrest, including intracranial hemorrhage or cerebrovascular accident, massive pulmonary emboli, pneumothorax, acute aortic dissection, and intra-abdominal hemorrhage is considered. If a non-coronary cause is not identified, then coronary angiography is performed with a target time of less than 2 hours from arrival, unless clear contraindications exist and PCI is performed when indicated. In patients with refractory VF, we use mechanical CPR with the LUCAS chest compression device (Physio-Control Inc.) to facilitate emergent transport from the field directly to the CCL. Patients who meet the criteria undergo emergent coronary angiography and PCI while ongoing CPR is performed. If ROSC is achieved after PCI, the patients are placed on hemodynamic support, if needed. Given the results of studies mentioned, we are working to develop an ECPR program at our hospital.

SUMMARY

OHCA and VF carries a high mortality rate, and is challenging to treat. Conventional therapies including early high-quality CPR, defibrillation, and optimal medical therapy remain the cornerstone of management. However, a significant proportion of these patients are refractory to conventional therapy. Recent trials evaluating novel therapies and strategies including early coronary angiography and ECPR have provided encouraging results.

SUPPLEMENTARY DATA

Supplementary data related to this article can be found online at https://doi.org/10.1016/j.ccl.2018.03.007.

REFERENCES

1. Benjamin EJ, Blaha MJ, Chiuve SE, et al. Heart disease and stroke statistics—2017 update: a report from the American Heart Association. Circulation 2017;135(10):e146–603.
2. Sakai T, Iwami T, Tasaki O, et al. Incidence and outcomes of out-of-hospital cardiac arrest with shock-resistant ventricular fibrillation: data from a large population-based cohort. Resuscitation 2010;81(8): 956–61.
3. Eifling M, Razavi M, Massumi A. The evaluation and management of electrical storm. Tex Heart Inst J 2011;38(2):111–21.
4. Vellano K, Crouch A, Rajdev M. Cardiac Arrest Registry to Enhance Survival (CARES)report on the public health burden of out-of-hospital cardiac arrest. 2015:19. Available at: https://mycares.net/sitepages/uploads/2015/CARES%20IOM%20Formatted.pdf. Accessed December 5, 2017.
5. Link MS, Berkow LC, Kudenchuk PJ, et al. Part 7: adult advanced cardiovascular life support: 2015 American Heart Association guidelines update for cardiopulmonary resuscitation and emergency cardiovascular care. Circulation 2015;132(18 suppl 2): S444–64.
6. Holmberg M, Holmberg S, Herlitz J. Incidence, duration and survival of ventricular fibrillation in

out-of-hospital cardiac arrest patients in Sweden. Resuscitation 2000;44(1):7–17.

7. Kragholm K, Wissenberg M, Mortensen RN, et al. Bystander efforts and 1-year outcomes in out-of-hospital cardiac arrest. N Engl J Med 2017; 376(18):1737–47.

8. Warden C, Cudnik MT, Sasson C, et al. Poisson cluster analysis of cardiac arrest incidence in Columbus, Ohio. Prehosp Emerg Care 2012;16(3):338–46.

9. Mitchell MJ, Stubbs BA, Eisenberg MS. Socioeconomic status is associated with provision of bystander cardiopulmonary resuscitation. Prehosp Emerg Care 2009;13(4):478–86.

10. Vaillancourt C, Lui A, De Maio VJ, et al. Socioeconomic status influences bystander CPR and survival rates for out-of-hospital cardiac arrest victims. Resuscitation 2008;79(3):417–23.

11. Sasson C, Haukoos JS, Eigel B, et al. The HANDDS program: a systematic approach for addressing disparities in the provision of bystander cardiopulmonary resuscitation. Acad Emerg Med 2014;21(9): 1042–9.

12. Adelborg K, Thim T, Secher N, et al. Benefits and shortcomings of mandatory first aid and basic life support courses for learner drivers. Resuscitation 2011;82(5):614–7.

13. Merchant RM, Abella BS, Abotsi EJ, et al. Cell phone cardiopulmonary resuscitation: audio instructions when needed by lay rescuers: a randomized, controlled trial. Ann Emerg Med 2010;55(6):538–43.e1.

14. Semeraro F, Taggi F, Tammaro G, et al. iCPR: a new application of high-quality cardiopulmonary resuscitation training. Resuscitation 2011;82(4):436–41.

15. Brooks SC, Anderson ML, Bruder E, et al. Part 6: alternative techniques and ancillary devices for cardiopulmonary resuscitation: 2015 American Heart Association Guidelines update for cardiopulmonary resuscitation and emergency cardiovascular care. Circulation 2015;132(18 suppl 2):S436–43.

16. Krarup NH, Terkelsen CJ, Johnsen SP, et al. Quality of cardiopulmonary resuscitation in out-of-hospital cardiac arrest is hampered by interruptions in chest compressions—a nationwide prospective feasibility study. Resuscitation 2011;82(3):263–9.

17. Perkins GD, Lall R, Quinn T, et al. Mechanical versus manual chest compression for out-of-hospital cardiac arrest (PARAMEDIC): a pragmatic, cluster randomised controlled trial. Lancet 2015;385(9972):947–55.

18. Rubertsson S, Lindgren E, Smekal D, et al. Mechanical chest compressions and simultaneous defibrillation vs conventional cardiopulmonary resuscitation in out-of-hospital cardiac arrest: the LINC randomized trial. JAMA 2014;311(1):53–61.

19. Hayashida K, Tagami T, Fukuda T, et al. Mechanical cardiopulmonary resuscitation and hospital survival among adult patients with nontraumatic out-of-hospital cardiac arrest attending the emergency department: a prospective, multicenter, observational study in Japan (SOS-KANTO [Survey of Survivors after Out-of-Hospital Cardiac Arrest in Kanto Area] 2012 Study). J Am Heart Assoc 2017;6(11): e007420.

20. Merlin MA, Tagore A, Bauter R, et al. A case series of double sequence defibrillation. Prehosp Emerg Care 2016;20(4):550–3.

21. Leacock BW. Double simultaneous defibrillators for refractory ventricular fibrillation. J Emerg Med 2014;46(4):472–4.

22. Jost D, Degrange H, Verret C, et al. DEFI 2005: a randomized controlled trial of the effect of automated external defibrillator cardiopulmonary resuscitation protocol on outcome from out-of-hospital cardiac arrest. Circulation 2010;121(14):1614–22.

23. Kudenchuk PJ, Cobb LA, Copass MK, et al. Amiodarone for resuscitation after out-of-hospital cardiac arrest due to ventricular fibrillation. N Engl J Med 1999;341(12):871–8.

24. Kudenchuk PJ, Brown SP, Daya M, et al. Amiodarone, lidocaine, or placebo in out-of-hospital cardiac arrest. N Engl J Med 2016;374(18):1711–22.

25. Overgaard CB, Džavík V. Inotropes and vasopressors: review of physiology and clinical use in cardiovascular disease. Circulation 2008;118(10): 1047–56.

26. Michael JR, Guerci AD, Koehler RC, et al. Mechanisms by which epinephrine augments cerebral and myocardial perfusion during cardiopulmonary resuscitation in dogs. Circulation 1984; 69(4):822–35.

27. Ewy GA, Bobrow BJ, Chikani V, et al. The time dependent association of adrenaline administration and survival from out-of-hospital cardiac arrest. Resuscitation 2015;96(Supplement C):180–5.

28. Ong ME, Tan EH, Ng FS, et al. Survival outcomes with the introduction of intravenous epinephrine in the management of out-of-hospital cardiac arrest. Ann Emerg Med 2007;50(6):635–42.

29. Jacobs IG, Finn JC, Jelinek GA, et al. Effect of adrenaline on survival in out-of-hospital cardiac arrest: a randomised double-blind placebo-controlled trial. Resuscitation 2011;82(9):1138–43.

30. Gueugniaud P-Y, Mols P, Goldstein P, et al. A comparison of repeated high doses and repeated standard doses of epinephrine for cardiac arrest outside the hospital. N Engl J Med 1998;339(22): 1595–601.

31. Brown CG, Martin DR, Pepe PE, et al. A comparison of standard-dose and high-dose epinephrine in cardiac arrest outside the hospital. N Engl J Med 1992; 327(15):1051–5.

32. Callaham M, Madsen CD, Barton CW, et al. A randomized clinical trial of high-dose epinephrine

and norepinephrine vs standard-dose epinephrine in prehospital cardiac arrest. JAMA 1992;268(19): 2667–72.

33. Bartos JA, Voicu S, Matsuura TR, et al. Role of epinephrine and extracorporeal membrane oxygenation in the management of ischemic refractory ventricular fibrillation: a randomized trial in pigs. JACC Basic Transl Sci 2017;2(3):244–53.

34. Mukoyama T, Kinoshita K, Nagao K, et al. Reduced effectiveness of vasopressin in repeated doses for patients undergoing prolonged cardiopulmonary resuscitation. Resuscitation 2009;80(7):755–61.

35. Tang W, Weil MH, Gazmuri RJ, et al. Pulmonary ventilation/perfusion defects induced by epinephrine during cardiopulmonary resuscitation. Circulation 1991;84(5):2101–7.

36. de Oliveira FC, Feitosa-Filho GS, Ritt LEF. Use of beta-blockers for the treatment of cardiac arrest due to ventricular fibrillation/pulseless ventricular tachycardia: a systematic review. Resuscitation 2012;83(6):674–83.

37. Driver BE, Debaty G, Plummer DW, et al. Use of esmolol after failure of standard cardiopulmonary resuscitation to treat patients with refractory ventricular fibrillation. Resuscitation 2014;85(10): 1337–41.

38. Dezfulian C, Shiva S, Alekseyenko A, et al. Nitrite therapy after cardiac arrest reduces reactive oxygen species generation, improves cardiac and neurological function, and enhances survival via reversible inhibition of mitochondrial complex I. Circulation 2009;120(10):897–905.

39. Dezfulian C, Alekseyenko A, Dave KR, et al. Nitrite therapy is neuroprotective and safe in cardiac arrest survivors. Nitric Oxide 2012;26(4):241–50.

40. Duranski MR, Greer JJM, Dejam A, et al. Cytoprotective effects of nitrite during in vivo ischemia-reperfusion of the heart and liver. J Clin Invest 2005;115(5):1232–40.

41. Dezfulian C, Olsufka M, Fly D, et al. Hemodynamic effects of IV sodium nitrite in hospitalized comatose survivors of out of hospital cardiac arrest. Resuscitation 2018;122(Supplement C):106–12.

42. Moulaert VRMP, Verbunt JA, van Heugten CM, et al. Cognitive impairments in survivors of out-of-hospital cardiac arrest: a systematic review. Resuscitation 2009;80(3):297–305.

43. Bernard SA, Gray TW, Buist MD, et al. Treatment of comatose survivors of out-of-hospital cardiac arrest with induced hypothermia. N Engl J Med 2002; 346(8):557–63.

44. Hypothermia after Cardiac Arrest Study Group. Mild therapeutic hypothermia to improve the neurologic outcome after cardiac arrest. N Engl J Med 2002; 346(8):549–56.

45. Nielsen N, Wetterslev J, Cronberg T, et al. Targeted temperature management at 33°C versus 36°C after cardiac arrest. N Engl J Med 2013; 369(23):2197–206.

46. Callaway CW, Donnino MW, Fink EL, et al. Part 8: post–cardiac arrest care: 2015 American Heart Association Guidelines update for cardiopulmonary resuscitation and emergency cardiovascular care. Circulation 2015;132(18 suppl 2):S465–82.

47. Kim F, Nichol G, Maynard C, et al. Effect of prehospital induction of mild hypothermia on survival and neurological status among adults with cardiac arrest: a randomized clinical trial. JAMA 2014;311(1): 45–52.

48. Chelly J, Mongardon N, Dumas F, et al. Benefit of an early and systematic imaging procedure after cardiac arrest: insights from the PROCAT (Parisian Region Out of Hospital Cardiac Arrest) registry. Resuscitation 2012;83(12):1444–50.

49. Spaulding CM, Joly L-M, Rosenberg A, et al. Immediate coronary angiography in survivors of out-of-hospital cardiac arrest. N Engl J Med 1997; 336(23):1629–33.

50. Lam DH, Glassmoyer LM, Strom JB, et al. Factors associated with performing urgent coronary angiography in out-of-hospital cardiac arrest patients. Catheter Cardiovasc Interv 2017. https://doi.org/10. 1002/ccd.27199.

51. Camuglia AC, Randhawa VK, Lavi S, et al. Cardiac catheterization is associated with superior outcomes for survivors of out of hospital cardiac arrest: review and meta-analysis. Resuscitation 2014;85(11):1533–40.

52. Kern KB, Lotun K, Patel N, et al. Outcomes of comatose cardiac arrest survivors with and without ST-segment elevation myocardial infarction: importance of coronary angiography. JACC Cardiovasc Interv 2015;8(8):1031–40.

53. Yannopoulos D, Bartos JA, Raveendran G, et al. Coronary artery disease in patients with out-of-hospital refractory ventricular fibrillation cardiac arrest. J Am Coll Cardiol 2017;70(9):1109–17.

54. Burrell AJC, Pellegrino VA, Wolfe R, et al. Long-term survival of adults with cardiogenic shock after venoarterial extracorporeal membrane oxygenation. J Crit Care 2015;30(5):949–56.

55. Riou B, Adnet F, Baud F, et al. Recommandations sur les indications de l'assistance circulatoire dans le traitement des arrêts cardiaques réfractaires. Ann Fr Anesth Réanim 2009;28(2):182–6.

56. Chen W-C, Huang K-Y, Yao C-W, et al. The modified SAVE score: predicting survival using urgent veno-arterial extracorporeal membrane oxygenation within 24 hours of arrival at the emergency department. Crit Care 2016;20(1):336.

57. Stub D, Bernard S, Pellegrino V, et al. Refractory cardiac arrest treated with mechanical CPR, hypothermia, ECMO and early reperfusion (the CHEER trial). Resuscitation 2015;86:88–94.

58. Belohlavek J, Kucera K, Jarkovsky J, et al. Hyperinvasive approach to out-of hospital cardiac arrest using mechanical chest compression device, prehospital intraarrest cooling, extracorporeal life support and early invasive assessment compared to standard of care. A randomized parallel groups comparative study proposal. "Prague OHCA study". J Transl Med 2012;10:163.

59. Chen Y-S, Chao A, Yu H-Y, et al. Analysis and results of prolonged resuscitation in cardiac arrest patients rescued by extracorporeal membrane oxygenation. J Am Coll Cardiol 2003;41(2):197–203.

60. Dorian P, Cass D, Schwartz B, et al. Amiodarone as compared with lidocaine for shock-resistant ventricular fibrillation. N Engl J Med 2002;346(12):884–90.

61. Tzivoni D, Banai S, Schuger C, et al. Treatment of torsade de pointes with magnesium sulfate. Circulation 1988;77(2):392–7.

62. Laurent I, Adrie C, Vinsonneau C, et al. High-volume hemofiltration after out-of-hospital cardiac arrest: a randomized study. J Am Coll Cardiol 2005;46(3): 432–7.

63. Bray JE, Stub D, Bloom JE, et al. Changing target temperature from 33°C to 36°C in the ICU management of out-of-hospital cardiac arrest: a before and after study. Resuscitation 2017;113(Suppl C):39–43.

64. Kämäräinen A, Virkkunen I, Tenhunen J, et al. Prehospital therapeutic hypothermia for comatose survivors of cardiac arrest: a randomized controlled trial. Acta Anaesthesiol Scand 2009;53(7):900–7.

The Role of Medical Direction in Systems of Out-of-Hospital Cardiac Arrest

Holbrook Hill Stoecklein, MD[a,b,*],
Scott T. Youngquist, MD, MS, FAEMS[a,b]

KEYWORDS

- Out-of-hospital cardiac arrest • EMS • Quality assurance • Medical direction

KEY POINTS

- The variability in observed survival rates for out-of-hospital cardiac arrest (OHCA) among emergency medical services (EMS) systems is largely due to differences in system performance rather than patient characteristics.
- Basic life support care during OHCA has the greatest impact on survival and should be the cornerstone of quality assessment of EMS system performance.
- Data collection and comparison used to target specific interventions, along with continuous feedback, shape the quality-assurance process and reduce variability.
- Process improvements can yield significant improvements in outcomes for OHCA, but these require the concentrated efforts and vision of a dedicated medical director.

BACKGROUND

Emergency medical services (EMS) are a vital part of the emergency and trauma care infrastructure in the United States. Dedicated men and women respond each day to more than 240 million calls for help received through a universal emergency response (9-1-1) telephone number.[1] And yet, EMS is still in its infancy, having only been established in the past 60 years through a piecemeal legislative and grant process involving federal, state, and private initiatives. Given the haphazard nature of EMS development and historic underappreciation of its role in the larger health care system, variability in the scope and quality of prehospital care have been such defining characteristics[2] as to inspire the saying, "If you've seen one EMS system, you've seen one EMS system." Approximately half of all EMS systems are fire-based, resulting in a sometimes uneasy alignment of modern prehospital care with the traditional paramilitary and rescue culture of the fire service. Other systems run as dedicated third service government programs (separate from police and fire), hospital-based services, or third-party contractors. Regardless of the type of EMS system involved, EMS medical directors play a vital role in assuring that the systems over which they have oversight adhere to the highest standards of medical care. A 2017 National Association of EMS Physicians position statement makes it clear that "The primary role of the EMS medical director is to promote continuous quality improvement and patient centered care delivery of medical care by

Disclosure: The authors have nothing to disclose.
a Salt Lake City Fire Department, University of Utah School of Medicine, Salt Lake City, UT, USA; b Division of Emergency Medicine, Department of Surgery, University of Utah, University of Utah School of Medicine, 30 North 1900 East, 1C026, Salt Lake City, UT 84132, USA
* Corresponding author. Division of Emergency Medicine, University of Utah School of Medicine, 30 North 1900 East, 1C026, Salt Lake City, UT 84132.
E-mail address: Hill.stoecklein@hsc.utah.edu

Cardiol Clin 36 (2018) 409–417
https://doi.org/10.1016/j.ccl.2018.03.008
0733-8651/18/© 2018 Elsevier Inc. All rights reserved.

the EMS service."[3] Unfortunately, in many communities the medical directorship of the local EMS agency is an unpaid position delegated to an untrained junior partner of a local emergency medicine physician group. Such positions often involve little more than titular duties: the "signing off" on protocols developed by subordinates or the making of ad hoc decisions as problems arise.[4]

IMPORTANCE

Of the many types of emergencies to which EMS personnel are dispatched, a minority (<5%) are for patients who have experienced out-of-hospital cardiac arrest (OHCA). Yet, although representing a small fraction of the annual call volume of an EMS agency, OHCA is a condition for which the quality of EMS care literally means the difference between life and death. More than 347,000 adults experience OHCA in the United States each year,[5] with an average survival of approximately 10%. But survival varies widely between communities, from a dismal less than or equal to 2% in some of the nation's largest municipalities[6-8] to 21% in Seattle, King County, Washington.[9] Differences in arrest characteristics, as summarized by the so-called Utstein elements, account for less than half of the observed variation in cardiac arrest survival and only 22% of the between-site differences in survival of bystander-witnessed arrests with an initial shockable rhythm,[10] all suggesting that EMS performance accounts for a large proportion of the disparity in outcomes.

GOALS OF THIS CONCEPT ARTICLE

The goals of this article are to explain the role of the EMS medical director in overseeing the quality of prehospital resuscitation of OHCA, to examine specific care parameters worthy of time and attention, and to review the quality-improvement process in OHCA.

THE MEDICAL DIRECTOR'S ROLE IN ASSURING QUALITY

It is worthwhile to conceptualize the medical director's role according to domains of control and influence (**Fig. 1**), a framework popularized by the organizational behavior expert, Stephen R. Covey.[11] For example, the medical director should have direct control over EMS protocols, training programs, and the collection, review, and dissemination of provider performance metrics. Although a medical director does not have direct control over the quality of post–cardiac arrest

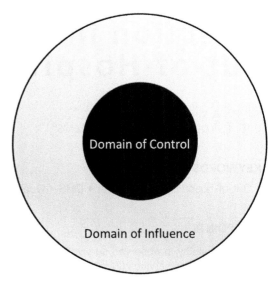

Fig. 1. A conceptual framework for the medical director's domains of control and influence in OHCA.

care delivered at receiving hospitals, the director often has influence over hospital destination protocols. These destination protocols should be informed by hospital capacity and performance characteristics, such as the willingness to provide EMS with feedback on patient outcomes, the performance of targeted temperature management for comatose patients, and the use of angiography for patients with shockable rhythms. In addition, the medical director can meet directly with heads of intensive care, emergency medicine, cardiology, and even the hospital chief executive officer in a collaborative fashion, ultimately exerting considerable influence over the quality of OHCA care across the care continuum.

DEFINING QUALITY IN CARDIOPULMONARY RESUSCITATION

Quality of care in cardiopulmonary resuscitation (CPR) may be measured by both process and outcomes. Processes of care center on EMS provider adherence to protocols because EMS provides protocol-driven medical care. Such protocols should be informed by international guidelines for basic life support (BLS) and advanced life support (ALS)[12] and tailored to the unique response configuration of the local EMS agency. Within guideline recommendations, considerable uncertainty exists regarding the optimal use and effectiveness of many ALS interventions (such as placement of an advanced airway). Nevertheless, these evidence-based guidelines, now updated nearly continuously, summarize the best available science in resuscitation and should be referred to when developing local protocols. The principal patient-oriented outcome of OHCA is survival to hospital discharge with good neurologic function. It is believed that improved care processes should ultimately result in improved outcomes from cardiac arrest. Communities that have adopted best practices from international guidelines, focusing on process quality, have measured such improved outcomes in OHCA.[13,14]

What Care Process Parameters Make a Difference?

The quality of BLS care in OHCA is of paramount importance[15–18] and it is BLS measures, for the most part, that have the greatest impact on survival and, thus, should be the focus of improvement (**Table 1**). The goal of achieving guidelines-compliant compression rate of 100 compressions/min to 120 compressions/min, depth of 2 in to 2.4 in, compression fraction of at least 80% (the percent of time during pulselessness when compressions are delivered), full chest release, and avoiding hyperventilation are low-hanging fruit for EMS quality improvement. These parameters are well informed by large-scale observational data including multiple studies from the Resuscitation Outcomes Consortium.[19–22] Unfortunately, full chest release cannot be measured without direct visual inspection. Chest compression release velocity, a

surrogate for chest recoil, is of uncertain value at this time.[23,24] For that reason, it is not included in quality reporting. Training crews to lift the palms of the hands off the sternum during the release phase of compressions is the only known method for reducing leaning.[25] Add to these parameters the timely and appropriate delivery of shocks to terminate ventricular fibrillation (VF) and pulseless ventricular tachycardia (VT)[18] and these 5 process parameters form reasonable, evidence-based benchmarks for field providers and the foundation of any resuscitation quality program. Poor compression quality, hyperventilation, and failure to deliver timely shocks should be considered avoidable medical errors.[26] Excellent ALS performance does not compensate for poor BLS care.

Dispatchers for 9-1-1 are a community's initial first responders and play a vital role in (1) rapidly identifying that a cardiac arrest has occurred, (2) quickly dispatching the closest available EMS crew, and (3) starting prearrival instructions, including the performance of dispatch-assisted CPR, sometimes called telephone CPR, and informing callers of the location of any nearby defibrillators.[27] A program for quality improvement for 9-1-1 dispatch can improve the rate of bystander CPR, reducing the period of no-flow during arrest.[28]

Cardiac Arrest Case Definition

Cardiac arrest is broadly defined to include all patients receiving either a shock from a bystander automated external defibrillator or chest compressions administered by EMS personnel. This reduces cases of syncope or altered level of consciousness where chest compressions by bystanders alone are followed by recovery. Cases of obvious drowning, strangulation, or traumatic arrest are excluded.

The Improvement Process

Four general stages of quality assurance and continuous improvement have been recognized: collection, comparison, targeted interventions, and feedback. In the setting of cardiac arrest quality assurance, the provision of feedback is inextricably part of the intervention and many steps in the process happen simultaneously. Nevertheless, the overall process happens in a repeated fashion so an endpoint is never reached and progress is always possible (**Fig. 2**). Correctly performed, the effort is able to, at once, move performance toward a goal while simultaneously reducing variability in performance, as symbolized by the process flow arrow in **Fig. 2**. The Seattle/King County Fire Department pioneered the use of audit

Table 1 Recommended basic life support and advanced life support data to be collected and evaluated as part of the quality-assurance process	
Basic Life Support Measures	**Advanced Life Support Measures**
Average compression rate of 100/min–120/min	Appropriate and timely defibrillation
Average compression depth of 2 in–2.4 in	Adherence to airway protocols
Chest compression fraction of at least 80%	Appropriate medication administration
Ventilation rate of 10 breaths/min	Appropriate duration of efforts
Use of automated external defibrillator	Appropriate field termination and transport decisions

The italicized BLS measures are considered foundational and of primary importance.

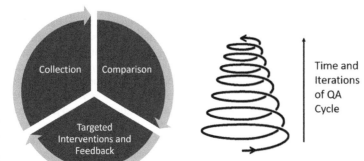

Fig. 2. Stages and development of the quality-assurance (QA) process.

and feedback to improve outcomes from cardiac arrest starting in the 1970s and has achieved worldwide recognition for outcomes from cardiac arrest that are among the very best. Seattle/King County's Dr Mickey Eisenberg's motto, "Measure and Improve, Measure and Improve," repeated endlessly, summarizes the process succinctly.

Data Collection

Collection of performance data in the modern era is facilitated by modern defibrillator technology that records chest compression data, the continuous ECG rhythm, end-tidal CO_2, and oxygen saturation as measured by pulse oximetry waveforms. Use of an accelerometer under the hands of providers allows for the real-time display and postincident review of compression rate, depth, and release velocity (the latter a surrogate for full chest release, which can only be monitored visually, otherwise). Because the defibrillator also displays real-time chest compression metrics, feedback begins as soon as chest compressions are initiated, creating the opportunity for immediate performance review by providers themselves. This instantaneous feedback occurs during data collection for offline review and improves performance before such formal review can take place.[29,30] Crews should be trained to orient the monitor so that providers performing compressions can monitor their own performance and make adjustments.

Some important observations can only be made by the medical director on the scene of a resuscitation attempt. For example, the medical director can directly assess team dynamics and observe the quality of field decision making. Yet there are potential drawbacks to this approach, aside from the commitment in time and resources to arrive on scene, including increased stress or performance anxiety on the part of providers and the potential to develop a biased estimate of the average quality of a resuscitation attempt in the system.

Nevertheless, field observation should be part of the overall approach to improving resuscitation quality.

After the incident, case files can usually be downloaded by hard line, wirelessly, or from cloud storage and directly attached to the electronic patient care report (ePCR). Each defibrillator manufacturer provides proprietary software from which summary reports of CPR quality can then be automatically generated. ALS cardiac monitors also allow providers to manually input code markers to label the timing of specific interventions. Time-stamped markers for the performance of intubation, medication administration, and manual pulse check results can be extremely useful during the review process but require training and feedback to implement. This is especially helpful given the known lack of accuracy of manual documentation for the timing of critical actions compared with events recorded directly on the monitor.[31] Case acquisition is facilitated by the use of an electronic health record for EMS incident documentation that allows for both broad and narrow search strategies. The authors search for primary or secondary impressions of cardiac arrest or respiratory arrest to identify possible cases. In agencies with limitations on manpower, it may be best to focus review only on those cases of bystander witnessed arrest presenting with an initial shockable rhythm, because this category of cardiac arrest has the highest survival potential.

Obtaining outcomes data from receiving hospitals can be challenging because misunderstandings concerning the scope and limitations of Health Insurance Portability and Accountability Act privacy protections abound. In Utah, the state's Clinical Health Information Exchange[32] is used to obtain outcomes when accurate identifying information is available at the time of EMS care. Hospital-EMS liaisons are relied on to obtain the rest. The State of Utah also participates in the Cardiac Arrest Registry to Enhance Survival, which was sponsored, in part, by the Centers for Disease

Control and Prevention in 2005 and now includes data from 36 states, more than 800 EMS agencies, and more than 100 cases per day.[33]

Data Comparison

Comparison of performance with guideline recommendations and written protocols is straightforward when the average rate and depth and chest compression fraction can be reported using manufacturer specific software. Although more time consuming, the authors also find it useful to record the longest pause observed during the case, the total number of pauses lasting greater than 10 seconds, the time from observation of a shockable rhythm to the delivery of a shock (with a target of, at most, every 2 minutes), and the duration of efforts when the resuscitation is terminated in the field. The ePCR is also reviewed to evaluate the appropriateness of ALS care regarding airway interventions, medication administration, and field termination or transport, as shown in **Table 1**.

Postincident Feedback

Postincident feedback is critical for improvement, training reinforcement, and encouraging buy-in from providers. The tone, source, and timing of feedback are equally important. Feedback is best received when it is nonpunitive and delivered with positive encouragement.[34] In fire-based systems, it is important to make clear that quality-improvement activities are exempt from consideration of promotion in rank. If concerning trends or reckless behavior are observed with individual providers, then these should be addressed individually and sometimes through a formal disciplinary process; otherwise, feedback should be provided to the entire crew under the assumption that today's missteps point the way to tomorrow's successes. Peer-to-peer performance review and feedback may be a useful model in some types of care, but in the setting of resuscitation performance the authors do not advise it, because it runs the risk of diluting the importance of cardiac arrest care if not guided by the medical director personally. If reviews are developed by subordinates, the medical director should review and finalize them before delivering feedback from the director's own email account or in person, with the latter the most impactful but often the least feasible in the context of a busy schedule. Critical errors should prompt direct medical director involvement in brief retraining exercises. Regardless of the mode of communication, a standardized form for reporting performance measures (**Fig. 3**) not only allows for data tracking at a system level but also serves to reinforce expectations in a standardized fashion.

Finally, the sooner after a patient care encounter feedback can be given, the more likely it is to have an impact on the providers involved.

DEFINING AND ADDRESSING CRITICAL ERRORS

When discussing the concept of error reduction in prehospital resuscitation, even when every link in the chain of survival is in place, the outcome is often still as if none of them was. In 2018, most patients still fail to respond to even the best care in the highest-performing EMS systems. It is perhaps worthwhile to consider then that critical errors in cardiac arrest do not directly "kill patients" but may, when repeated, substantially reduce the likelihood of survival in the population.

Two simple categories of errors exist: failures to act (omission) and the performance of actions that are potentially harmful (commission). **Fig. 4** is an example of a failure to act in which a paramedic misclassified the cardiac rhythm as asystole throughout the resuscitation attempt. Based on this misclassification, he failed to deliver a shock to treat the true rhythm, VF, and resuscitative efforts were ultimately terminated in the field. VF was later easily identified by the medical director in postincident review. The medical director then met with the paramedic, who was able to identify the rhythm as VF when challenged after the fact and could not account for the misinterpretation on scene. This type of critical cognitive error would never have come to light without postincident review. The literature is sparse regarding the accuracy of paramedic rhythm interpretation for VF versus asystole. Pirrallo and colleagues,[35] however, using tabletop exercises, found that paramedic agreement on VF is amplitude-dependent and that the lower the VF waveform amplitude, the greater the likelihood that the rhythm is misclassified as asystole. To address the real potential for this critical cognitive error, the authors adopted a protocol of administering an empiric shock to patients initially classified as a rhythm of asystole after 2 to 3 rounds of chest compressions as a system-level failsafe.

On the other hand, errors of improper action often result from external circumstances affecting individual performance, such as fatigue and interruptions during task performance. Effective team structure, including adoption of a pit crew–style resuscitation in which participants are focused on a limited number of decision points and tasks, the use of checklists, and scene control to minimize interruptions or distractions can mitigate this type of error. An example is adoption of a verbal 10-second countdown from the provider performing compressions for any pause in CPR so

SLCFD Cardiac Arrest Care Standards

Incident Number:
Receiving Hospital:
Date of Service:

	Performed	Comments
Dispatch Assisted CPR		
Was the need for DACPR identified?		
Time from call receipt to recognition		
Were DACPR instructions provided?		
If instructions not given, reason?		
Defibrillation		
VF/VT shocked within 2 min		
Organized rhythm not shocked		
<10 s preshock pause		
CPR		
Rate of 110/min		
Depth 2–2.4 in		
Compression Fraction >80%		
Pauses <10 s		
Airway		
30:2 comp:vent ratio until advanced airway		
BVM only if age<14		
End-tidal CO2		
No hyperventilation (10 breaths/min)		
Other		
Code Markers Used		
Limit Scene Time for: ECMO, pregnancy, hypothermia		
Medications		
Antiarrhythmic for recurrent/refractory VF >3 shocks		
Glucose if hypoglycemic		
Bicarbonate only if suspected hyperkalemia		
Post-Arrest Care		
12 Lead ECG		
Transport to STEMI receiving center		
Maintain ETCO2 of 35–45 mm Hg		
Field Termination		
All criteria met: Not witnessed by EMS, no shock delivered (for VF/VT), no ROSC		
Called UUMC to review termination algorithm		
Appropriate duration of resuscitation: Asystole 30 min, otherwise 40 min		

Fig. 3. Example of a cardiac arrest care standards checklist. SLCFD, salt lake city fire department; DACPR, dispatch assisted cardiopulmonary resuscitation; BVM, bag valve mask; ECMO, extracorporeal membrane oxygenation; ETCO2, end-tidal carbon dioxide; ROSC, return of spontaneous circulation; STEMI, ST-elevation myocardial infarction; UUMC, University of Utah Medical Center.

the entire team is aware of pause duration which is easy to lose track of when numerous other interventions or tasks are being performed.

After understanding the types of errors that are possible in a system, defining a relative hierarchy of errors may help in deciding how to prioritize interventions aimed at correcting errors when multiple errors are observed. This hierarchy may be system-specific but should be based on the knowledge of which interventions are known to

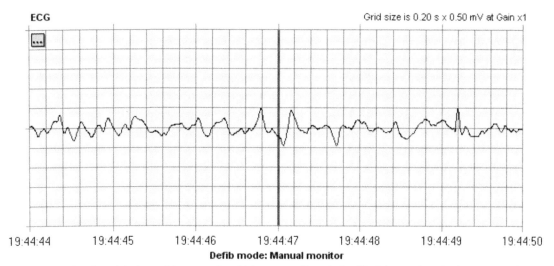

Fig. 4. Example of a critical cognitive error in which paramedics misclassified the cardiac rhythm as asystole and failed to administer a shock. Defib mode is monitor notation for defibrillation mode.

have the greatest impact on survival for OHCA. As an example, a protocol deviation with misuse of lidocaine instead of amiodarone for refractory VF, therapies that evidence has shown to be equivalent,[36] is considered a less significant error than failure to defibrillate that same patient with refractory VF. A general suggestion for a hierarchy of errors specific to OHCA is included in **Box 1**.

IMPROVEMENTS IN OUTCOMES FOLLOW IMPROVEMENTS IN PROCESS

In the authors' system, a multifaceted restructuring of approach to cardiac arrest care, including emphasis on high-quality CPR with real-time and postincident feedback, adoption of a pit crew

---

Box 1
Hierarchy of errors in out-of-hospital cardiac arrest based on the likelihood of impact on survival

Critical errors

No defibrillation of a shockable rhythm

Inappropriate field termination of resuscitation

Major errors

Compression pauses greater than 10 seconds

Hyperventilation

Compression depth too deep, too shallow, or without full recoil

Minor errors

Medication errors

Deviations from airway protocol

---

approach to resuscitation, simplification of protocols based on clinical evidence and updated guidelines, and implementation of a more robust QA process resulted in a rate of neurologically intact survival almost twice as high for OHCA patients in the postintervention group.[14] Other investigators have observed similar results.[13,30,37,38] Such improvements require the guiding vision and force of an engaged EMS medical director. The American Heart Association, HeartRescue Project,[39] and Take Heart America[40] all provide valuable resources to medical directors interested in improving outcomes from cardiac arrest and are a great starting point for learning more.

SUMMARY

EMS medical directors play a vital role in assuring the quality of care for OHCA victims. With modern technology, it is now easier than ever to track both the processes and outcomes of prehospital cardiac arrest care in a manner that is evidence-based and limits critical errors. System progress still requires, however, the dedication of a medical director's own human capital to achieve system-level improvements. A focus on the BLS aspects of resuscitation—high-quality chest compressions and rapid defibrillation—should be the foundation of any oversight program. The future survival of cardiac arrest victims depends on it.

REFERENCES

1. 9-1-1 Statistics-National Emergency Number Association. Available at: https://www.nena.org/?page= 911Statistics. Accessed December 28, 2017.

2. Institute of Medicine. Emergency medical services: at the crossroads. Washington, DC: National Academies Press; 2007.

3. Physician oversight of emergency medical services. Prehosp Emerg Care 2017;21(2):281–2.

4. Greer S, Williams I, Valderrama AL, et al. EMS medical direction and prehospital practices for acute cardiovascular events. Prehosp Emerg Care 2013;17(1):38–45.

5. Benjamin EJ, Blaha MJ, Chiuve SE, et al. Heart disease and stroke statistics—2017 update: a report from the American Heart Association. Circulation 2017;135(10):e146–603.

6. Eckstein M, Stratton SJ, Chan LS. Cardiac arrest resuscitation evaluation in Los Angeles: CARE-LA. Ann Emerg Med 2005;45(5):504–9.

7. Becker LB, Ostrander MP, Barrett J, et al. Outcome of CPR in a large metropolitan area–where are the survivors? Ann Emerg Med 1991;20(4):355–61.

8. Westfal RE, Reissman S, Doering G. Out-of-hospital cardiac arrests: an 8-year New York City experience. Am J Emerg Med 1996;14(4):364–8.

9. Zive D, Koprowicz K, Schmidt T, et al. Variation in out-of-hospital cardiac arrest resuscitation and transport practices in the resuscitation outcomes consortium: ROC Epistry–Cardiac arrest. Resuscitation 2011;82(3):277–84.

10. Rea TD, Cook AJ, Stiell IG, et al. Predicting survival after out-of-hospital cardiac arrest: role of the Utstein data elements. Ann Emerg Med 2010;55(3):249–57.

11. Covey SR. The 7 habits of highly effective people: powerful lessons in personal change. 25th anniversary edition. New York: Simon & Schuster; 2013.

12. Olasveengen TM, de Caen AR, Mancini ME, et al. 2017 International consensus on cardiopulmonary resuscitation and emergency cardiovascular care science with treatment recommendations summary. Circulation 2017;136(23):e424–40.

13. Kudenchuk PJ, Redshaw JD, Stubbs BA, et al. Impact of changes in resuscitation practice on survival and neurological outcome after out-of-hospital cardiac arrest resulting from nonshockable arrhythmias. Circulation 2012;125(14):1787–94.

14. Hopkins CL, Burk C, Moser S, et al. Implementation of pit crew approach and cardiopulmonary resuscitation metrics for out-of-hospital cardiac arrest improves patient survival and neurological outcome. J Am Heart Assoc 2016;5(1). https://doi.org/10.1161/JAHA.115.002892.

15. Stiell IG, Wells GA, Field B, et al. Advanced cardiac life support in out-of-hospital cardiac arrest. N Engl J Med 2004;351(7):647–56.

16. Cournoyer A, Notebaert É, Iseppon M, et al. Prehospital advanced cardiac life support for out-of-hospital cardiac arrest: a cohort study. Acad Emerg Med 2017;24(9):1100–9.

17. Sanghavi P, Jena AB, Newhouse JP, et al. Outcomes after out-of-hospital cardiac arrest treated by basic vs advanced life support. JAMA Intern Med 2015;175(2):196.

18. Valenzuela TD, Roe DJ, Nichol G, et al. Outcomes of rapid defibrillation by security officers after cardiac arrest in casinos. N Engl J Med 2000;343(17):1206–9.

19. Stiell IG, Brown SP, Nichol G, et al. What is the optimal chest compression depth during out-of-hospital cardiac arrest resuscitation of adult patients? Circulation 2014;130(22):1962–70.

20. Idris AH, Guffey D, Pepe PE, et al. Chest compression rates and survival following out-of-hospital cardiac arrest. Crit Care Med 2015;43(4):840–8.

21. Christenson J, Andrusiek D, Everson-Stewart S, et al. Chest compression fraction determines survival in patients with out-of-hospital ventricular fibrillation. Circulation 2009;120(13):1241–7.

22. Indik JH, Conover Z, McGovern M, et al. Amplitude-spectral area and chest compression release velocity independently predict hospital discharge and good neurological outcome in ventricular fibrillation out-of-hospital cardiac arrest. Resuscitation 2015;92:122–8.

23. Cheskes S, Common MR, Byers AP, et al. The association between chest compression release velocity and outcomes from out-of-hospital cardiac arrest. Resuscitation 2015;86:38–43.

24. Kovacs A, Vadeboncoeur TF, Stolz U, et al. Chest compression release velocity: association with survival and favorable neurologic outcome after out-of-hospital cardiac arrest. Resuscitation 2015;92:107–14.

25. Aufderheide TP, Pirrallo RG, Yannopoulos D, et al. Incomplete chest wall decompression: a clinical evaluation of CPR performance by EMS personnel and assessment of alternative manual chest compression-decompression techniques. Resuscitation 2005;64(3):353–62.

26. Meaney PA, Bobrow BJ, Mancini ME, et al. Cardiopulmonary resuscitation quality: improving cardiac resuscitation outcomes both inside and outside the hospital: a consensus statement from the American Heart Association. Circulation 2013;128(4):417–35.

27. Ornato JP. Performance goals for dispatcher-assisted cardiopulmonary resuscitation. Circulation 2013;128(14):1490–1.

28. Bohm K, Vaillancourt C, Charette ML, et al. In patients with out-of-hospital cardiac arrest, does the provision of dispatch cardiopulmonary resuscitation instructions as opposed to no instructions improve outcome: a systematic review of the literature. Resuscitation 2011;82(12):1490–5.

29. Hostler D, Everson-Stewart S, Rea TD, et al. Effect of real-time feedback during cardiopulmonary resuscitation outside hospital: prospective, cluster-randomised trial. BMJ 2011;342:d512.

30. Kramer-Johansen J, Myklebust H, Wik L, et al. Quality of out-of-hospital cardiopulmonary resuscitation with real time automated feedback: a prospective interventional study. Resuscitation 2006;71(3):283–92.

31. Frisch A, Reynolds JC, Condle J, et al. Documentation discrepancies of time-dependent critical events in out of hospital cardiac arrest. Resuscitation 2014; 85(8):1111–4.

32. UHIN | The cHIE's data sources. Available at: https://uhin.org/the-chies-data-sources/. Accessed January 1, 2018.

33. About CARES «MyCares. Available at: https://mycares.net/sitepages/aboutcares.jsp. Accessed December 31, 2017.

34. Foerster CR, Tavares W, Virkkunen I, et al. A survey of front-line paramedics examining the professional relationship between paramedics and physician medical oversight. CJEM 2017;1–9. https://doi.org/10.1017/cem.2017.36.

35. Pirrallo RG, Swor RA, Maio RF. Inter-rater agreement of paramedic rhythm labeling. Ann Emerg Med 1993;22(11):1684–7.

36. Kudenchuk PJ, Brown SP, Daya M, et al. Amiodarone, lidocaine, or placebo in out-of-hospital cardiac arrest. N Engl J Med 2016;374(18): 1711–22.

37. Lund-Kordahl I, Olasveengen TM, Lorem T, et al. Improving outcome after out-of-hospital cardiac arrest by strengthening weak links of the local chain of survival; quality of advanced life support and post-resuscitation care. Resuscitation 2010;81(4): 422–6.

38. Bleijenberg E, Koster RW, de Vries H, et al. The impact of post-resuscitation feedback for paramedics on the quality of cardiopulmonary resuscitation. Resuscitation 2017;110:1–5.

39. Home. Heart Rescue Project. Available at: http://www.heartrescueproject.com/. Accessed January 2, 2018.

40. Take Heart America – The cutting edge approach to improve cardiac arrest survival. Available at: http://takeheartamerica.org/. Accessed January 2, 2018.

Critical Care of the Post–Cardiac Arrest Patient

Amy C. Walker, MD[a], Nicholas J. Johnson, MD[a,b],*

KEYWORDS

- Cardiac arrest • Critical care • Postarrest • Return of spontaneous circulation
- Out-of-hospital cardiac arrest • ROSC • Post–cardiac arrest syndrome

KEY POINTS

- The post–cardiac arrest syndrome is a highly inflammatory state characterized by organ dysfunction, ischemia and reperfusion injury, and persistent precipitating pathology.
- Patients with ST-elevation myocardial infarction or high suspicion for cardiac etiology should undergo early coronary angiography.
- Multiple trials have shown that active temperature management after cardiac arrest, regardless of rhythm, results in improved outcome.
- After cardiac arrest, arterial oxygen and carbon dioxide tensions should be normalized immediately, and patients should be ventilated with low tidal volumes.
- The optimal approach to neurologic prognostication is multimodal, combining clinical examination with diagnostic tests, no sooner than 72 hours to 96 hours after cardiac arrest.

INTRODUCTION

Sudden cardiac arrest affects more than 500,000 people in the United States each year. Patients who achieve return of spontaneous circulation (ROSC) after cardiac arrest often represent the extreme of critical illness. Severe ischemia-reperfusion injury often results in damage to multiple organ systems, which evolves even after resuscitation. Several postarrest critical care interventions improve outcome by addressing underlying precipitating pathology, restoring normal perfusion to damaged organs, and limiting the effects of ischemia-reperfusion injury. This article reviews the pathophysiology of the post–cardiac arrest state and discusses several critical care interventions aimed at improving outcome for patients after ROSC (**Fig. 1**).

THE POST–CARDIAC ARREST SYNDROME

Following ROSC after cardiac arrest, many patients suffer from the post–cardiac arrest syndrome (PCAS), which includes 4 components: (1) brain injury, (2) myocardial dysfunction, (3) systemic ischemia and reperfusion injury, and (4) persistent precipitating pathology.[1]

Brain injury after cardiac arrest is complex, with underlying pathophysiology that involves excitotoxicity, abnormal calcium homeostasis, free radical formation, pathologic protease cascades, and activation of apoptotic pathways.[1] Many of these pathways are activated in the hours to days after ROSC. Additional insults, such as hypotension, hypoxemia, pyrexia, dysglycemia, and seizures, can be extremely damaging.

The PCAS is most notably characterized by profound ischemia-reperfusion injury. Because

Disclosure: N.J. Johnson receives funding from the National Institutes of Health (U01HL123008-02) and Medic One Foundation. A.C. Walker has nothing to disclose.
[a] Department of Emergency Medicine, University of Washington, Harborview Medical Center, 325 9th Avenue, Box 359702, Seattle, WA 98104, USA; [b] Division of Pulmonary, Critical Care, and Sleep Medicine, University of Washington, Harborview Medical Center, 325 9th Avenue, Box 359702, Seattle, WA 98104, USA
* Corresponding author. Department of Emergency Medicine, University of Washington, Harborview Medical Center, 325 9th Avenue, Box 359702, Seattle, WA 98104.
E-mail address: nickj45@uw.edu

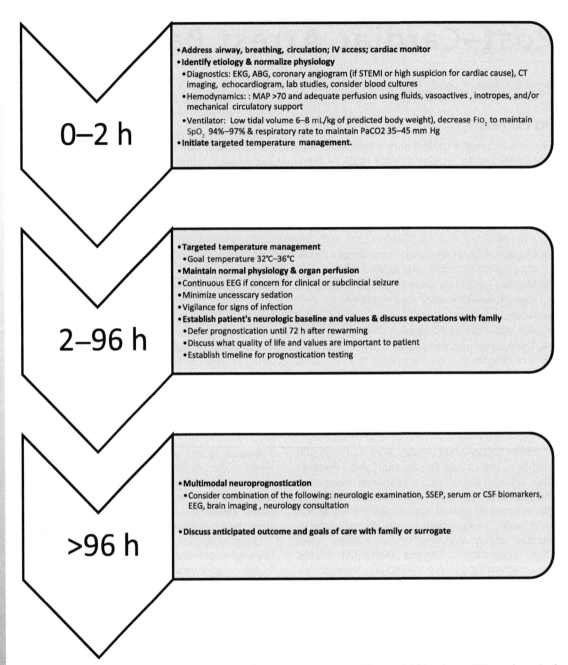

0–2 h
- Address airway, breathing, circulation; IV access; cardiac monitor
- Identify etiology & normalize physiology
  - Diagnostics: EKG, ABG, coronary angiogram (if STEMI or high suspicion for cardiac cause), CT imaging, echocardiogram, lab studies, consider blood cultures
  - Hemodynamics:: MAP >70 and adequate perfusion using fluids, vasoactives, inotropes, and/or mechanical circulatory support
  - Ventilator: Low tidal volume 6–8 mL/kg of predicted body weight), decrease F_{IO_2} to maintain SpO_2 94%–97% & respiratory rate to maintain PaCO2 35–45 mm Hg
- Initiate targeted temperature management.

2–96 h
- Targeted temperature management
  - Goal temperature 32°C–36°C
- Maintain normal physiology & organ perfusion
- Continuous EEG if concern for clinical or subclincial seizure
- Minimize uncesscary sedation
- Vigilance for signs of infection
- Establish patient's neurologic baseline and values & discuss expectations with family
  - Defer prognostication until 72 h after rewarming
  - Discuss what quality of life and values are important to patient
  - Establish timeline for prognostication testing

>96 h
- Multimodal neuroprognostication
  - Consider combination of the following: neurologic examination, SSEP, serum or CSF biomarkers, EEG, brain imaging, neurology consultation
- Discuss anticipated outcome and goals of care with family or surrogate

Fig. 1. Timeline of key post–cardiac arrest critical care interventions. ABG, arterial blood gas; CSF, cerebrospinal fluid; EKG, electrocardiogram; IV, intravenous; PEEP, positive end-expiratory pressure; SSEP, somatosensory evoked potentials.

cardiac arrest is the extreme of shock states, oxygen delivery is dramatically reduced during the arrest event, leading to profound tissue hypoxia. Prolonged ischemia also leads to buildup of reactive oxygen species in tissues that are then distributed widely on reperfusion. Tissue hypoxia causes inflammation and microvascular thrombosis, which contribute to multiorgan dysfunction.

Finally, if the underlying pathology that caused the initial cardiac arrest is not addressed, then ongoing injury to the brain and other organs is likely during the vulnerable postarrest period. Diagnosis of underlying precipitating conditions, such as acute coronary syndrome, can be challenging given the complex pathophysiological state of the PCAS.

IDENTIFYING AND ADDRESSING ETIOLOGY

Identifying the etiology of cardiac arrest allows for tailored medical therapy and interventions targeting the underlying condition. All patients should receive an ECG immediately after ROSC to assess for ST-segment elevation myocardial infarction (STEMI).

Coronary Angiography

Current guidelines recommend immediate coronary angiography (CAG) for all patients with STEMI on postarrest ECG and suspected cardiac origin.[2] Although entirely observational, existing data suggest that early CAG for patients without a clear noncardiac cause is associated with improved outcome, especially in patients with an initial shockable rhythm.[3–7] Several studies suggest that there may be benefit to early percutaneous coronary intervention for all patients with an initial shockable rhythm but are potentially limited by selection bias.[3,6,8,9] In the era of public reporting of percutaneous coronary intervention outcomes, physicians may be less likely to offer CAG for critically ill patients, in particular those who are likely to have worse outcomes.[10,11] A recent guideline recommends early CAG for patients without STEMI on ECG, provided the following factors are absent: a noncardiac cause or unfavorable resuscitation features.[12]

Identifying Noncardiac Etiology

It is estimated that 70% to 85% of out-of-hospital cardiac arrest (OHCA) cases are cardiac in etiology.[13] Noncardiac causes include neurologic, respiratory, trauma, toxic and metabolic. In pulseless electrical activity (PEA) specifically, ECG intervals have been found to correlate with etiology of arrest. Narrow complex PEA may be more likely to represent mechanical cause of arrest (eg, hypovolemia, tension pneumothorax, or tamponade), whereas wide complex PEA more commonly suggests metabolic derangements, such as hyperkalemia or acidemia.[14]

There is likely an important role for imaging in the undifferentiated PCAS patient. Subarachnoid hemorrhage is a potential cause for OHCA and may be associated with ST-segment changes on ECG. Although the incidence in European populations is believed low, the incidence in East Asian populations is as high as 25%.[7,15–17] Imaging directed at other diagnoses, such as pulmonary embolism, aortic dissection, infection, and hemorrhagic shock, should be considered based on the clinical circumstance if no alternate etiology is found.

TEMPERATURE MANAGEMENT

After multiple preclinical studies, 2 landmark clinical trials demonstrated that treatment with induced mild therapeutic hypothermia improved neurologic outcome after OHCA[18,19] (**Table 1**). Bernard and colleagues[18] randomized patients with ventricular fibrillation (VF) or ventricular tachycardia (VT) OHCA to receive therapeutic hypothermia at 33°C or normothermia for 12 hours. They demonstrated an improvement from 26% to 49% in neurologically intact survival to hospital discharge among the 43 patients treated with therapeutic hypothermia.

Table 1
Summary of targeted temperature management randomized trials

Study	Temperatures	Arrest Rhythm	No. of Patients	Primary Outcome
Bernard et al,[18] 2002	33°C vs normal	VT/VF	77	Neurointact survival to discharge 49% vs 26[a]
HACA,[19] 2002	32°C–34°C vs normal	VT/VF	273	Neurointact survival at 6 mo 55% vs 39%[a]
Kim et al,[30] 2014	Prehospital cooling vs usual care	VT/VF PEA Asystole	1359	Survival and neuro status at discharge No difference
Nielsen et al,[29] 2014	33°C vs 36°C	VT/VF PEA Asystole	939	All-cause mortality at 90 d 50% vs 48
Kirkegaard et al,[31] 2017	33°C × 24 h vs 33°C × 48 h	VT/VF PEA Asystole	355	Neurointact survival at 6 mo 69% vs 64%

[a] Indicates a statistically significant difference.

Similarly, the Hypothermia After Cardiac Arrest (HACA) investigators randomized 273 patients with VT/VF OHCA to therapeutic hypothermia (32°C –34°C) or normothermia for 24 hours postarrest and found a 16% improvement in neurologically intact survival at 6 months.[19] Taken together, these trials informed wide adoption of therapeutic hypothermia and inclusion in international guidelines. Subsequent observational studies of temperature management demonstrated variable results in different patient populations, including in-hospital cardiac arrest and nonshockable rhythms.[20–26] Two pediatric randomized trials examining the impact of therapeutic hypothermia to 33°C for in-hospital and OHCA, respectively, demonstrated no survival benefit or difference in neurologic outcome at 1 year.[27,28]

Nielsen and colleagues[29] published a large, multicenter trial in which 939 patients with OHCA with a presumed cardiac etiology were randomized to a goal temperature of 33°C or 36°C. No difference was found in their primary outcome of all-cause mortality at 90 days, and few significant differences were demonstrated in multiple subgroup analyses. Patients randomized to 33°C had a greater requirement for support with vasoactive or inotropic agents and had more electrolyte derangements. A randomized trial by Kim and colleagues[30] found no benefit when cooling was initiated in the prehospital setting. A recent trial found no difference between targeted temperature management (TTM) to 33°C for 24 hours versus 48 hours.[31]

Guidelines have afforded some clinicians some flexibility, recommending active temperature management targeting a goal temperature of 32°C to 36°C for all comatose survivors of cardiac arrest.[2] Although many institutions have changed their protocols to target 36°C, there have been reports of worsened outcomes at this higher target temperature.[32,33] A study comparing 33°C to controlled normothermia is in progress (NCT02908308).

RESPIRATORY CARE
Oxygenation

Preclinical studies found that reducing the fraction of inspired oxygen (FIO_2) after cardiac arrest decreases neuronal injury and oxidative stress.[34–36] Clinical studies have demonstrated mixed results. A retrospective analysis of more than 6000 patients in a large critical care database found that PaO_2 greater than or equal to 300 mm Hg was associated with an 18% absolute increase in hospital mortality compared with patients who were maintained within the normal range.[37] Hypoxemia was associated with a similarly poor outcome. The same group demonstrated that each 100–mm Hg increase in PaO_2 was associated with a 24% increase in risk of death, implying a dose-dependent relationship.[38] Subsequent observational studies have yielded conflicting results.[39–44]

Several randomized trials have been performed. A small pilot study randomized patients after OHCA to rapid titration of FIO_2 in the prehospital setting to maintain oxygen saturation as measured by pulse oximetry (SpO_2) of 90% to 94% or standard oxygen therapy to maintain SpO_2 greater than 95%. The study was stopped with just 17 patients enrolled after 7 of 8 patients in the titrated oxygen group achieved a prespecified safety endpoint of SpO_2 less than 88%.[45] The Oxygen-ICU trial randomized all-comers admitted to a single ICU to conservative (PaO_2 70–100 mm Hg or SpO_2 94%–98%) versus standard (PaO_2 <150 mm Hg or SpO_2 97%–100%) oxygen therapy on ICU admission.[46] In 434 randomized patients, the conservative oxygen therapy group had lower PaO_2 values (87 vs 102 mm Hg) and mortality (12 vs 20%) compared with the standard group.[47] Whether a similar effect would be seen among postarrest patients is unknown.

Current guidelines recommend titration of FIO_2 to maintain SpO_2 greater than or equal to 94%.[2] Because of the potential risk posed by hyperoxemia, the authors suggest immediate titration of FIO_2 to maintain SpO_2 94% to 97% as soon as feasible, which correlates approximately with PaO_2 70 mm Hg to 100 mm Hg, along with early arterial blood gas analysis (**Table 2**).

Ventilation

The relationship between ventilation, partial pressure of arterial carbon dioxide ($PaCO_2$), and outcome after cardiac arrest is complex. Hyperventilation during cardiac arrest is known to cause poor coronary and cerebral perfusion, owing to

Table 2 Recommendations for respiratory parameters after cardiac arrest	
Oxygenation	SpO_2 94%–97% PaO_2 70 mm Hg–100 mm Hg Positive end-expiratory pressure $\geq$5 cm H_2O
Ventilation	$PaCO_2$ 40 mm Hg–45 mm Hg If ARDS, tidal volume: 4 mL/kg–6 mL/kg of predicted body weight If no ARDS, tidal volume $\leq$8 mL/kg of predicted body weight

increased intrathoracic pressure leading to lower venous return.[48] After cardiac arrest, abnormalities in $Paco_2$ may affect cerebral blood flow and worsen secondary ischemic injury. Numerous observational studies have examined the association between $Paco_2$ and outcome.[41,49–52] Because the studies used a variety of definitions and blood gas sampling time periods, reported results are variable. Arterial hypocarbia has fairly consistently been associated with poor neurologic outcome after cardiac arrest, but the relationship between hypercarbia and neurologic outcome is less clear.[41,49–52] A systematic review and meta-analysis that included 8 studies and 23,000 patients demonstrated that normocarbia was associated with favorable neurologic outcome compared with both hypercarbia and hypocarbia.[53] In a pilot trial, 86 patients who suffered OHCA were randomized to mild hypercarbia ($Paco_2$ of 50–55 mm Hg) or normocarbia ($Paco_2$ of 35–45 mm Hg) for 24 hours after hospital admission.[54] Patients randomized to mild hypercarbia had lower serum concentrations of biomarkers of neurologic injury and a nonsignificant trend toward favorable neurologic outcome.

Guidelines recommend $Paco_2$ be maintained within the normal range of 35 mm Hg to 45 mm Hg after cardiac arrest[2] (see **Table 2**). Mild permissive hypercarbia is an experimental strategy that warrants further study. Early blood gas analysis should be performed after ROSC, because prescribed minute ventilation and end-tidal CO_2 values correlate poorly with $Paco_2$.[51,55,56]

Infection, Lung Injury, and the Acute Respiratory Distress Syndrome

Patients who suffer from the PCAS often develop immune dysregulation, making them more susceptible to infection.[57–59] Several series report incidences of infection of up to 70%, with the respiratory tract and bloodstream the most common sources.[60–62] Diagnosis of infection is particularly challenging in the PCAS population, because many patients have evidence of systemic inflammation, and traditional triggers for infectious work-ups, such as fever, are masked by TTM. For patients with aspiration, the authors recommend early sampling of the lower respiratory tract and empiric antimicrobials until cultures are negative.[63]

Patients who suffer cardiac arrest are also at risk for the acute respiratory distress syndrome (ARDS). Potential risk factors include aspiration, infection, pulmonary contusion due to chest compressions, and reperfusion injury. Although the epidemiology of ARDS after cardiac arrest has not yet been well characterized, 1 study demonstrated that approximately 65% of PCAS patients had a Pao_2:Fio_2 ratio less than or equal to 300, consistent with the hypoxemia criterion in the Berlin Definition of ARDS.[64,65] Low tidal volume ventilation applied to patients with ARDS led to a 9% absolute decrease in mortality, and observational data suggest that ventilation with lower tidal volumes may be associated with fewer pulmonary complications in patients without ARDS.[66,67] A propensity-matched cohort study demonstrated an association between lower tidal volumes (defined as ≤8 mL/kg of predicted body weight) and favorable neurologic status in 256 patients who suffered OHCA.[68]

In summary, clinicians should aggressively search for infection and consider empiric treatment in high-risk patients with PCAS. Clinicians should treat postarrest patients who meet the definition of ARDS using a low-tidal volume strategy and consider such a strategy even in PCAS patients without ARDS (see **Table 2**).

HEMODYNAMICS

Given the propensity for hemodynamic lability and the sensitivity of the brain to additional ischemia after cardiac arrest, careful hemodynamic monitoring is essential. The authors recommend invasive arterial blood pressure monitoring and central venous access for comatose cardiac arrest survivors with evidence of hemodynamic compromise. Pulmonary artery catheters and cardiac output monitoring may be considered but have not been shown to improve outcome.[2] The authors also recommend early echocardiography to assess for myocardial dysfunction. It is reasonable to trend mean arterial pressure (MAP), lactate and other laboratory markers of organ function, urine output, and central venous oxygen saturation.

The optimal blood pressure goal after cardiac arrest is not known, but hypotension after cardiac arrest is an independent predictor of mortality and should be avoided.[69–71] Several observational studies have demonstrated association between higher MAP goals and improved outcome, even if those goals are achieved with vasopressors.[72–74] A randomized trial assessing the effect of higher MAP on brain injury after cardiac arrest is under way (NCT02541591).[74]

The approach to resuscitation should be individualized based on a patient's physiology. One retrospective study compared patients with postarrest shock who were resuscitated with high fluid volume (>700 mL) and low dose of vasopressors to those receiving high-dose vasopressors and low fluid volume. The authors demonstrated improved outcome in the high fluid volume and low-dose vasopressor group, but potential for confounding based on underlying physiology exists.[75] In patients with refractory cardiogenic shock, mechanical circulatory support may be indicated.

In summary, hypotension should be avoided after cardiac arrest and may be corrected by volume resuscitation, vasopressors, inotropes, and mechanical support based on a patient's underlying physiology. Observational data suggest that higher MAPs may be beneficial, but further prospective study is needed.

PROGNOSTICATION

Withdrawal of life-sustaining therapy (WLST) is the most common cause of death for patients admitted after OHCA.[76] Accurate prognostication is, therefore, imperative. Most prognostication tools offer insight into which patients are likely to have poor neurologic recovery, whereas few tools help clinicians predict who will awaken (**Table 3**).

Timing

The earliest time for prognostication based on clinical examination findings should be 72 hours after rewarming for patients who undergo TTM and 72 hours after arrest for those not undergoing TTM.[2] A retrospective study found that approximately 15% of patients discharged with a favorable neurologic outcome after OCHA had delayed awakening, suggesting that a nontrivial proportion of patients may still awaken greater

Table 3
Summary of prognostication tools

Prognostication Tool	Description	Estimated False-Positive Rate[2]
Clinical examination • Pupillary reflex • Corneal reflex • Motor response • Myoclonus	• All may be affected by TTM, sedatives, and paralytics. • Absent bilateral pupillary reflex at 72 h is highly specific for poor neurologic outcome (0%FPR). • Absent motor response and extensor posturing has high FPR in the setting of TTM (up to 15%). • Status myoclonus, (continuous, repetitive myoclonic jerks lasting more than 30 min) is associated with poor prognosis.	0%–15%
Electroencephalogram • Burst suppression • Absent reactivity during and after TTM • Status epilepticus	• Existing data are variable in quality. • EEG may be most useful for detecting subclinical seizures.	0%–2%
Somatosensory evoked potentials	• Assesses cortical response to repetitive peripheral nerve stimulation. • Believed less affected by sedation and TTM than EEG and motor examination	1%–2%
Biomarkers • S-100 • Neuron-specific enolase	• High levels of S-100 in the first 24 h and serial neuron-specific enolase levels increasing over 72 h have each been shown to correlate with poor neurologic outcome. • No cutoff value has been identified to reliably predict poor outcome.	No cutoff identified
Imaging • CT • MRI	• Reduced gray-white matter ratio on CT and apparent diffusion coefficient and diffusion-weighted imaging abnormalities on MRI are all markers of edema on which has been correlated with poor neurologic outcome	0%–8%

Abbreviations: FPR, false-positive rate; S-100B, S-100 calcium-binding protein B.
Data from Callaway CW, Donnino MW, Fink EL, et al. Part 8: post-cardiac arrest care: 2015 American Heart Association guidelines update for cardiopulmonary resuscitation and emergency cardiovascular care. Circulation 2015;132(18):S465–82.

than 72 hours after rewarming.[77] In a propensity-matched retrospective study, Elmer and colleagues[78] estimated that 16% of the patients with early WLST might have had good neurologic recovery.[78]

Multimodal Approach

A multimodal approach to determining neurologic prognosis for patients who are comatose after OHCA is recommended, although there is no perfect formula. The authors recommend using a combination of physical examination, continuous electroencephalography (EEG), and at least 1 of the following to confirm poor prognosis prior to consideration of WLST: somatosensory evoked potentials, biomarkers, or neuroimaging[2] (see **Table 3**). If data are equivocal, further testing and imaging should be pursued and should be interpreted in the context of a patient's preexisting functional status and values.

SUMMARY

Critical care after cardiac arrest should focus on restoring normal physiology, limiting further injury, and optimizing neurologic outcome. Key aspects include identifying and addressing etiology, restoring adequate hemodynamics and organ perfusion, TTM, maintenance of normal oxygen and carbon dioxide tensions and prevention of lung injury, and multimodal prognostication (see **Fig. 1**).

REFERENCES

1. Neumar RW, Nolan JP. Post-cardiac arrest syndrome. Circulation 2008;118:2452–83.
2. Callaway CW, Donnino MW, Fink EL, et al. Part 8: post-cardiac arrest care: 2015 American Heart Association guidelines update for cardiopulmonary resuscitation and emergency cardiovascular care. Circulation 2015;132(18):S465–82.
3. Dumas F, Bougouin W, Geri G, et al. Emergency percutaneous coronary intervention in post–cardiac arrest patients without st-segment elevation pattern. JACC Cardiovasc Interv 2016;9(10):1011–8.
4. Dumas F, Cariou A, Manzo-Silberman S, et al. Immediate percutaneous coronary intervention is associated with better survival after out-of-hospital cardiac arrest: insights from the PROCAT (Parisian Region Out of Hospital Cardiac Arrest) registry. Circ Cardiovasc Interv 2010;3(3):200–7.
5. Reynolds JC, Callaway CW, El Khoudary SR, et al. Coronary angiography predicts improved outcome following cardiac arrest: propensity-adjusted analysis. J Intensive Care Med 2007; 24(3):179–86.
6. Vyas A, Chan PS, Cram P, et al. Early coronary angiography and survival after out-of-hospital cardiac arrest. Circ Cardiovasc Interv 2015;8(10):e002321.
7. Kim Y-J, Min S-Y, Lee DH, et al. The role of post-resuscitation electrocardiogram in patients with st-segment changes in the immediate post-cardiac arrest period. JACC Cardiovasc Interv 2017;10(5): 451–9.
8. Cronier P, Vignon P, Bouferrache K, et al. Impact of routine percutaneous coronary intervention after out-of-hospital cardiac arrest due to ventricular fibrillation. Crit Care 2011;15:R122.
9. Martínez-Losas P, Salinas P, Ferrera C, et al. Coronary angiography findings in cardiac arrest patients with non-diagnostic post-resuscitation electrocardiogram: a comparison of shockable and non-shockable initial rhythms. World J Cardiol 2017; 9(8):702.
10. Peberdy MA, Donnino MW, Callaway CW, et al. Impact of percutaneous coronary intervention performance reporting on cardiac resuscitation centers: a scientific statement from the American Heart Association. Circulation 2013;128(7):762–73.
11. McCabe JM, Joynt KE, Welt FGP, et al. Impact of public reporting and outlier status identification on percutaneous coronary intervention case selection in Massachusetts. JACC Cardiovasc Interv 2013; 6(6):625–30.
12. Rab T, Kern KB, Tamis-Holland JE, et al. Cardiac arrest: a treatment algorithm for emergent invasive cardiac procedures in the resuscitated comatose patient. J Am Coll Cardiol 2015;66(1):62–73.
13. McNally B, Robb R, Mehta M, et al. Out-of-hospital cardiac arrest surveillance — Cardiac Arrest Registry to Enhance Survival (CARES), United States, October 1, 2005–December 31, 2010. MMWR Surveill Summ 2011;60(8):1–19.
14. Littmann L, Bustin DJ, Haley MW. A simplified and structured teaching tool for the evaluation and management of pulseless electrical activity. Med Princ Pract 2014;23(1):1–6.
15. Skrifvars MB, Parr MJ. Incidence, predisposing factors, management and survival following cardiac arrest due to subarachnoid haemorrhage: a review of the literature. Scand J Trauma Resusc Emerg Med 2012;20(1):75.
16. Arnaout M, Mongardon N, Deye N, et al. Out-of-hospital cardiac arrest from brain cause. Crit Care Med 2015;43(2):453–60.
17. Inamasu J, Miyatake S, Tomioka H, et al. Subarachnoid haemorrhage as a cause of out-of-hospital cardiac arrest: a prospective computed tomography study. Resuscitation 2009;80(9):977–80.
18. Bernard SA, Gray TW, Buist MD, et al. Treatment of comatose survivors of out-of-hospital cardiac arrest with induced hypothermia. N Engl J Med 2002; 346(8):557–63.

19. Hypothermia After Cardiac Arrest (HACA) Study Group. Mild therapeutic hypothermia to improve the neurologic outcome after cardiac arrest. N Engl J Med 2002;346(8):549–56.

20. Don CW, Longstreth WT, Maynard C, et al. Active surface cooling protocol to induce mild therapeutic hypothermia after out-of-hospital cardiac arrest: a retrospective before-and-after comparison in a single hospital. Crit Care Med 2009;37(12):3062–9.

21. Dumas F, Grimaldi D, Zuber B, et al. Is hypothermia after cardiac arrest effective in both shockable and nonshockable patients?: Insights from a large registry. Circulation 2011;123(8):877–86.

22. Kim YM, Yim HW, Jeong SH, et al. Does therapeutic hypothermia benefit adult cardiac arrest patients presenting with non-shockable initial rhythms?: A systematic review and meta-analysis of randomized and non-randomized studies. Resuscitation 2012; 83(2):188–96.

23. Perman SM, Grossestreuer AV, Wiebe DJ, et al. The utility of therapeutic hypothermia for post-cardiac arrest syndrome patients with an initial nonshockable rhythm. Circulation 2015;132(22):2146–51.

24. Testori C, Sterz F, Behringer W, et al. Mild therapeutic hypothermia is associated with favourable outcome in patients after cardiac arrest with non-shockable rhythms. Resuscitation 2011;82(9): 1162–7.

25. Dankiewicz J, Schmidbauer S, Nielsen N, et al. Safety, feasibility, and outcomes of induced hypothermia therapy following in-hospital cardiac arrest-evaluation of a large prospective registry. Crit Care Med 2014;42(12):2537–45.

26. Nichol G, Huszti E, Kim F, et al. Does induction of hypothermia improve outcomes after in-hospital cardiac arrest? Resuscitation 2013;84(5):620–5.

27. Moler FW, Silverstein FS, Holubkov R, et al. Therapeutic hypothermia after out-of-hospital cardiac arrest in children. N Engl J Med 2015;372(20): 1898–908.

28. Moler FW, Silverstein FS, Holubkov R, et al. Therapeutic hypothermia after in-hospital cardiac arrest in children. N Engl J Med 2017;376(4):318–29.

29. Nielsen N, Wetterslev J, Cronberg T, et al. Targeted temperature management at 33°C versus 36°C after cardiac arrest. N Engl J Med 2013;369(23): 2197–206.

30. Kim F, Nichol G, Maynard C, et al. Effect of prehospital induction of mild hypothermia on survival and neurological status among adults with cardiac arrest: a randomized clinical trial. JAMA 2014;311(1): 45–52.

31. Kirkegaard H, Søreide E, de Haas I, et al. Targeted temperature management for 48 vs 24 hours and neurologic outcome after out-of-hospital cardiac arrest. JAMA 2017;318(4):341.

32. Deye N, Vincent F, Michel P, et al. Changes in cardiac arrest patients' temperature management after the 2013 "TTM" trial: results from an international survey. Ann Intensive Care 2016;6(1):4.

33. Bray JE, Stub D, Bloom JE, et al. Changing target temperature from 33C to 36C in the ICU management of out-of-hospital cardiac arrest: a before and after study. Resuscitation 2017;113:39–43.

34. Balan IS, Fiskum G, Hazelton J, et al. Oximetry-guided reoxygenation improves neurological outcome after experimental cardiac arrest. Stroke 2006;37(12):3008–13.

35. Vereczki V, Martin E, Rosenthal RE, et al. Normoxic resuscitation after cardiac arrest protects against hippocampal oxidative stress, metabolic dysfunction, and neuronal death. J Cereb Blood Flow Metab 2006;26(6):821–35.

36. Angelos MG, Yeh ST, Aune SE. Post-cardiac arrest hyperoxia and mitochondrial function. Resuscitation 2011;82:S48–51.

37. Kilgannon JH, Jones AE, Shapiro NI, et al. Association between arterial hyperoxia following resuscitation from cardiac arrest and in-hospital mortality. JAMA 2010;303(21):2165–71.

38. Kilgannon JH, Jones AE, Parrillo JE, et al. Relationship between supranormal oxygen tension and outcome after resuscitation from cardiac arrest. Circulation 2011;123:2717–22.

39. Janz DR, Hollenbeck RD, Pollock JS, et al. Hyperoxia is associated with increased mortality in patients treated with mild therapeutic hypothermia after sudden cardiac arrest. Crit Care Med 2013; 40(12):3135–9.

40. Ferguson LP, Durward A, Tibby SM. Relationship between arterial partial oxygen pressure after resuscitation from cardiac arrest and mortality in children. Circulation 2012;126:335–42.

41. Vaahersalo J, Bendel S, Reinikainen M, et al. Arterial blood gas tensions after resuscitation from out-of-hospital cardiac arrest: associations with long-term neurologic outcome. Crit Care Med 2014;42(6):1–8.

42. Bennett KS, Clark AE, Meert KL, et al. Early oxygenation and ventilation measurements after pediatric cardiac arrest: lack of association with outcome. Crit Care Med 2013;41(6):1534–42.

43. Bellomo R, Bailey M, Eastwood GM, et al. Arterial hyperoxia and in-hospital mortality after resuscitation from cardiac arrest. Crit Care 2011;15(2):R90.

44. Johnson NJ, Dodampahala K, Rosselot B, et al. The association between arterial oxygen tension and neurological outcome after cardiac arrest. Ther Hypothermia Temp Manag 2017;7(1):36–41.

45. Young P, Bailey M, Bellomo R, et al. HyperOxic therapy or normoxic therapy after out-of-hospital cardiac arrest (HOT OR NOT): a randomised controlled feasibility trial. Resuscitation 2014; 85(12):1686–91.

46. Eastwood GM, Tanaka A, Espinoza EDV, et al. Conservative oxygen therapy in mechanically ventilated patients following cardiac arrest: a retrospective nested cohort study. Resuscitation 2016; 101:108–14.

47. Girardis M, Busani S, Damiani E, et al. Effect of conservative vs conventional oxygen therapy on mortality among patients in an intensive care unit: the Oxygen-ICU randomized clinical trial. Jama 2016; 316(15):1583–9.

48. Aufderheide TP, Lurie KG. Death by hyperventilation: a common and life-threatening problem during cardiopulmonary resuscitation. Crit Care Med 2004; 32(9):S345–51.

49. Roberts BW, Kilgannon JH, Chansky ME, et al. Association between postresuscitation partial pressure of arterial carbon dioxide and neurological outcome in patients with post-cardiac arrest syndrome. Circulation 2013;127(21):2107–13.

50. Helmerhorst HJF, Roos-Blom MJ, van Westerloo DJ, et al. Associations of arterial carbon dioxide and arterial oxygen concentrations with hospital mortality after resuscitation from cardiac arrest. Crit Care 2015;19(1):348.

51. Tolins ML, Henning DJ, Gaieski DF, et al. Initial arterial carbon dioxide tension is associated with neurological outcome after resuscitation from cardiac arrest. Resuscitation 2017;114:53–8.

52. Wang C-H, Huang C-H, Chang W-T, et al. Association between early arterial blood gas tensions and neurological outcome in adult patients following in-hospital cardiac arrest. Resuscitation 2015;89:1–7.

53. McKenzie N, Williams TA, Tohira H, et al. A systematic review and meta-analysis of the association between arterial carbon dioxide tension and outcomes after cardiac arrest. Resuscitation 2017; 111:116–26.

54. Eastwood GM, Schneider AG, Suzuki S, et al. Targeted therapeutic mild hypercapnia after cardiac arrest: a phase II multi-centre randomised controlled trial (the CCC trial). Resuscitation 2016;104:83–90.

55. Roberts BW, Kilgannon JH, Chansky ME, et al. Association between initial prescribed minute ventilation and post-resuscitation partial pressure of arterial carbon dioxide in patients with post-cardiac arrest syndrome. Ann Intensive Care 2014;4(1):9.

56. Moon S-W, Lee S-W, Choi S-H, et al. Arterial minus end-tidal CO2 as a prognostic factor of hospital survival in patients resuscitated from cardiac arrest. Resuscitation 2007;72(2):219–25.

57. Adrie C, Adib-Conquy M, Laurent I, et al. Successful cardiopulmonary resuscitation after cardiac arrest as a "sepsis-like" syndrome. Circulation 2002;106: 562–8.

58. Bottiger BW, Motsch J, Bohrer H, et al. Activation of blood coagulation after cardiac arrest is not balanced adequately by activation of endogenous fibrinolysis. Circulation 1995;92(9):2572–8.

59. Neumar RW, Nolan JP, Adrie C, et al. Post-cardiac arrest syndrome: epidemiology, pathophysiology, treatment, and prognostication. A consensus statement from the international Liaison Committee on resuscitation (American Heart Association, Australian and New Zealand Council on Resuscitation. Circulation 2008;118(23):2452–83.

60. Mongardon N, Perbet S, Lemiale V, et al. Infectious complications in out-of-hospital cardiac arrest patients in the therapeutic hypothermia era. Crit Care Med 2011;39(6):1359–64.

61. Gaussorgues P, Gueugniaud PY, Vedrinne JM, et al. Bacteremia following cardiac arrest and cardiopulmonary resuscitation. Intensive Care Med 1988; 14(5):575–7.

62. Tsai MS, Chiang WC, Lee CC, et al. Infections in the survivors of out-of-hospital cardiac arrest in the first 7 days. Intensive Care Med 2005;31(5):621–6.

63. Ribaric SF, Turel M, Knafelj R, et al. Prophylactic versus clinically-driven antibiotics in comatose survivors of out-of-hospital cardiac arrest???A randomized pilot study. Resuscitation 2017;111:103–9.

64. Elmer J, Wang B, Melhem S, et al. Exposure to high concentrations of inspired oxygen does not worsen lung injury after cardiac arrest. Crit Care 2015;19:105.

65. Ranieri VM, Rubenfeld GD, Thompson BT, et al. Acute respiratory distress syndrome: the Berlin Definition. JAMA 2012;307(23):2526–33.

66. Acute Respiratory Distress Syndrome Network, Brower RG, Matthay MA, Morris A, et al. Ventilation with lower tidal volumes as compared with traditional tidal volumes for acute lung injury and the acute respiratory distress syndrome. N Engl J Med 2000;342: 1301–8.

67. Serpa Neto A, Nagtzaam L, Schultz MJ. Ventilation with lower tidal volumes for critically ill patients without the acute respiratory distress syndrome: a systematic translational review and meta-analysis. Curr Opin Crit Care 2014;20(1):25–32.

68. Beitler JR, Ghafouri TB, Joshua J. Favorable neurocognitive outcome with low tidal volume ventilation after cardiac arrest. Am J Respir Crit Care Med 2017;195(9):1198–206.

69. Chiu YK, Lui CT, Tsui KL. Impact of hypotension after return of spontaneous circulation on survival in patients of out-of-hospital cardiac arrest. Am J Emerg Med 2017;36(1):79–83.

70. Kilgannon JH, Roberts BW, Reihl LR, et al. Early arterial hypotension is common in the post-cardiac arrest syndrome and associated with increased in-hospital mortality. Resuscitation 2008;79(3):410–6.

71. Trzeciak S, Jones AE, Kilgannon JH, et al. Significance of arterial hypotension after resuscitation

from cardiac arrest. Crit Care Med 2009;37(11): 2895–903 [quiz: 2904].

72. Beylin ME, Perman SM, Abella BS, et al. Higher mean arterial pressure with or without vasoactive agents is associated with increased survival and better neurological outcomes in comatose survivors of cardiac arrest. Intensive Care Med 2013;39(11): 1981–8.

73. Kilgannon JH, Roberts BW, Jones AE, et al. Arterial blood pressure and neurologic outcome after resuscitation from cardiac arrest*. Crit Care Med 2014; 42(9):2083–91.

74. Ameloot K, De Deyne C, Ferdinande B, et al. Mean arterial pressure of 65 mm Hg versus 85-100 mm Hg in comatose survivors after cardiac arrest: rationale and study design of the Neuroprotect post–cardiac arrest trial. Am Heart J 2017;191:91–8.

75. Janiczek JA, Winger DG, Coppler P, et al. Hemodynamic resuscitation characteristics associated with improved survival and shock resolution after cardiac arrest. Shock 2016;45(6):613–9.

76. Elmer J, Rittenberger JC, Coppler PJ, et al. Long-term survival benefit from treatment at a specialty center after cardiac arrest. Resuscitation 2016;108: 48–53.

77. Zanyk-McLean K, Sawyer KN, Paternoster R, et al. Time to awakening is often delayed in patients who receive targeted temperature management after cardiac arrest. Ther Hypothermia Temp Manag 2017;7(2):95–100.

78. Elmer J, Torres C, Aufderheide TP, et al. Association of early withdrawal of life-sustaining therapy for perceived neurological prognosis with mortality after cardiac arrest. Resuscitation 2016;102:127–35.

Emerging and Future Technologies in Out-of-Hospital Cardiac Arrest Care

Andrew J. Latimer, MD[a],*, Andrew M. McCoy, MD, MS[a],
Michael R. Sayre, MD[b,c]

KEYWORDS

- Emergency medical services • Out-of-hospital cardiac arrest
- Extracorporeal membrane oxygenation • Ultrasound • Mobile applications • Aircraft • Defibrillators
- Crowdsourcing

KEY POINTS

- The management of victims of out-of-hospital cardiac arrest is rapidly evolving and new and emerging technologies will play a role in improving survival.
- The progression of extracorporeal life support and point-of-care ultrasound technologies both in-hospital and out-of-hospital may improve out-of-hospital cardiac arrest survival for certain subsets of patients.
- Unmanned aerial vehicles capable of delivering automated external defibrillators to the scene of a cardiac arrest may augment the available of early defibrillation by bystanders in some systems.
- Digital and mobile technologies to leverage bystander response could result in the next great leap in survival for victims of out-of-hospital cardiac arrest.

INTRODUCTION

Throughout history, the care for victims of out-of-hospital cardiac arrest (OHCA) has progressed through long periods of little advancement in knowledge separated by relatively brief periods of rapid advancements in the science. Modern human interests in resuscitating victims of sudden cardiac death began in the enlightenment era and slowly grew throughout the 18th and 19th centuries, principally in the port cities of Western Europe in response to the large number of victims of drowning and submersion injury.[1] These interests progressed to the creation of organizations interested in the care and resuscitation of victims of sudden death, namely the Amsterdam Rescue Society in the Netherlands and the Royal London Humane society in 1767 and 1774, respectively (**Fig. 1**). The creation of these societies arguably represents the first great step in the advancement of cardiac arrest science.

OHCA care again progressed rapidly and dramatically over the last half of the 20th century with the advent of closed chest cardiac massage and external cardiac defibrillation. The first case of successful closed chest cardiac massage was described in 1960[2] and was rapidly combined with mouth-to-mouth ventilation into modern day cardiopulmonary resuscitation (CPR), which was endorsed by the American Heart Association in 1963.[3] The first use of a portable external cardiac defibrillator was reported in 1967,[4] allowing for

Disclosure: The authors have nothing to disclose.
[a] Department of Emergency Medicine, University of Washington, Box 359702, 325 Ninth Avenue, Seattle, WA 98104-2499, USA; [b] Department of Emergency Medicine, University of Washington, Box 359727, 325 Ninth Avenue, Seattle, WA 98104-2499, USA; [c] Seattle Fire Department, Box 359702, 325 Ninth Avenue, Seattle, WA 98104-2499, USA
* Corresponding author.
E-mail address: alatim@uw.edu

Cardiol Clin 36 (2018) 429–441
https://doi.org/10.1016/j.ccl.2018.03.010
0733-8651/18/© 2018 Elsevier Inc. All rights reserved.

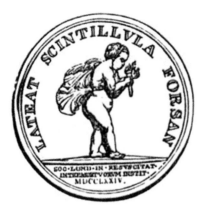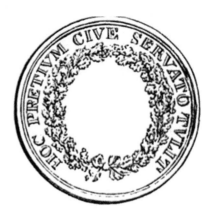

Fig. 1. The emblem of the Royal London Humane Society, founded in 1774. This token was given to those who were credited for assisting a person in distress. The front reads, "Lateat scintillula forsan" (A small spark may perhaps lie hid) and the back reads, "Hoc pretium cive servato tulit" (He has obtained this reward for having saved the life of a citizen). (*From* The Royal Humane Society. In: Newnes G, editor. The project Gutenberg ebook of the strand magazine, vol. V, Issue 28, 1893. Project Gutenberg; 2007. Available at: http://www.gutenberg.org/ebooks/20798. Accessed November 8, 2017.)

mobile treatments for victims of OHCA. Since that time, an array of technologies have been introduced that have improved the care of patients in OHCA, including portable and public access automatic external defibrillator (AED) technology, advanced computerized mathematical analysis of cardiac waveforms, mechanical CPR devices, and digital strategies to leverage bystander response. To this day, however, victims of OHCA have a relatively poor prognosis, even in the best of systems.[5]

There are a number of emerging therapeutics and technologies for the treatment of patients suffering from OHCA that may play an important role in the future of OHCA management, ranging from prehospital extracorporeal membranous oxygenation (ECMO), prehospital ultrasound imaging to improve the quality of CPR, automated flying drones to deliver AEDs directly to the scene of an OHCA, to digital and portable technologies for lay people that can detect cardiac arrest and notify good Samaritan bystanders as well as emergency medical services (EMS). One or several of these advances in combination may represent the next great leap in improving survival for patients of OHCA. In this article, we discuss some of these emerging and future technologies.

EXTRACORPOREAL MEMBRANOUS OXYGENATION AND APPLICATIONS FOR VICTIMS OF OUT-OF-HOSPITAL CARDIAC ARREST

There are roughly 365,000 OHCA events annually in the United States with an estimated survival rate of approximately 9%. This survival rate is highly variable from system to system, with reports ranging between 3% and 22%[5,6] of all prehospital treated cardiac arrests. Most patients that are successfully resuscitated with meaningful neurologic outcomes regain pulses by roughly minute 15 or by the third defibrillation attempt if the patient is in a shockable rhythm.[7] There are very few survivors of OHCA with favorable neurologic outcome receiving chest compressions for more than 45 minutes.[8]

It is challenging for prehospital providers to perform high-quality CPR during patient movement and transport,[9] and consistent high-quality closed chest CPR is correlated with survival.[10–13] Given these data, and in light of provider safety issues, many prehospital agencies in the United States have protocols that stress remaining on scene to complete the initial and critical resuscitation attempts for most patients suffering OHCA. Despite no current evidence demonstrating that mechanical CPR devices are more efficacious than manual CPR,[14–17] these devices may have a role in transporting certain cases of refractory cardiac arrest to the hospital.[18] There could be a subset of patients suffering from refractory cardiac arrest that may be successfully resuscitated if the underlying cause of the arrest, such as an occluded coronary artery, can be effectively addressed with advanced diagnostics and therapeutics only available in the hospital. Identifying this cohort, however, is challenging. Most hospitals currently do not have these therapies to offer a victim of refractory OHCA actively undergoing CPR.

An obstructed coronary artery is felt to be the cause of refractory cardiac arrest in as many as 80% of patients with an initial shockable rhythm that fail to be successfully resuscitated in the field.[19–21] These patients may benefit from the restoration of coronary blood flow during resuscitation. Some tertiary care centers have experimented with cardiac catheterization in a subset of patients in refractory ventricular fibrillation or pulseless ventricular tachycardia actively undergoing CPR and have had occasional success.[22–24] Emergent percutaneous coronary intervention is technically challenging while undergoing CPR; many patients with an acute coronary artery occlusion require significant hemodynamic support after percutaneous coronary intervention and do not regain sufficient cardiac output immediately after the procedure to survive. Many other patients in refractory cardiac arrest, specifically those in pulseless electrical activity or asystole, have an underlying etiology for their arrest other than occluded coronary arteries, including massive pulmonary embolism, poisoning, or environmental hypothermia. Interventions to address these pathologies are often not feasible while undergoing CPR.

Venoarterial ECMO, first invented in 1966, involves the placement of large arterial and venous catheters in line with a mechanical oxygenation and pump device that removes carbon dioxide, oxygenates blood, and maintains flows that can be similar to native cardiac output.[25] Venoarterial ECMO has become integrated into the hospital-based resuscitation of victims of cardiac arrest in some specialty centers over the last decade.[26,27] Using venoarterial ECMO in refractory cardiac arrest patients is often referred to as extracorporeal cardiac life support (ECLS). The advent of smaller and more affordable ECMO devices has allowed these specialty centers, in coordination with multidisciplinary teams, to use ECLS on patients in refractory cardiac arrest in the emergency department or the cardiac catheterization laboratory.[26,27]

The concept behind ECLS is to establish a perfusing cardiac output to allow time for providers to discover the precipitating cause of the refractory cardiac arrest and to allow intervention that would otherwise not be possible owing to the time and logistical constraints of a patient undergoing external chest compressions. Animal studies have suggested this approach may be superior to continuing standard Advanced Cardiac Life Support.[28] Several systems, both domestic and international, have had success in implementing ECLS for patients who have suffered OHCA refractory to traditional resuscitation attempts in the setting of an initially shockable rhythm with data reporting survival rates with favorable neurologic outcomes between 14% and 54%[29–33] (**Fig. 2**). Most of these patients

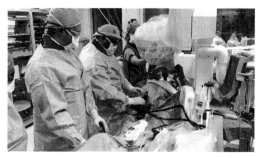

Fig. 2. Dr Demetris Yannopoulos and his team cannulating for extracorporeal cardiopulmonary resuscitation on a patient undergoing mechanical cardiopulmonary resuscitation in their cardiac catheterization laboratory at the University of Minnesota. (*Courtesy of* Demetris Yannopoulos, MD, Minneapolis, MN.)

would have died without this technology. Most of the patients with refractory ventricular fibrillation or pulseless ventricular tachycardia had a coronary occlusion that was amenable to intervention after the patient was supported with ECLS.[34]

PREHOSPITAL EXTRACORPOREAL MEMBRANOUS OXYGENATION

The current experience with ECLS in OHCA victims suggests that the time from collapse to ECMO flow is inversely correlated with survival and survival with favorable neurologic outcome.[29–31,33,34] These studies describe a substantial drop-off in survivors when the collapse to ECMO pump flow time exceeds 40 minutes. The logistics of EMS arriving on scene, attempting initial resuscitation of the cardiac arrest patient, identifying patients who would potentially benefit from ECLS, transporting these patients to a center capable of ECLS undergoing active resuscitation, and executing the in-hospital cannulation process within these time limits is challenging. Balancing traditional gold standard on-scene resuscitation for the majority of patients that are rapidly resuscitated with identifying those that are ECPR candidates and transporting them to the hospital in the appropriate time window creates a conundrum for EMS systems. Some data suggest that this time window for consideration of transport to maximize benefits of on-scene resuscitation versus time to ECPR cannulation on appropriate patients may lie around minute 15 of resuscitation; however, more research is needed.[35] In many systems, and in many specific patient scenarios, such as extrication from a tall building or large public spaces, achieving collapse to ECMO pump flow for in-hospital ECLS for the OHCA victim is not feasible in less than 60 minutes.[36,37]

Some systems have tried to shorten the time of CPR by bringing the ECMO pump and cannulation team to the patient. This step eliminates the need to transport the patient undergoing active CPR and, depending on the system model, can reduce the collapse to ECMO pump flow time.[37] The prehospital application of ECMO has been demonstrated by the Service d'Aide Médicale Urgente (SAMU) in France[38] (**Fig. 3**). The experience of this system uses the activation of a specialty physician-led prehospital team that performs out-of-hospital ECLS on victims of OHCA at the scene.[34,37–40] In a small cohort, SAMU has demonstrated that it is feasible to successfully perform prehospital ECMO cannulation for ECLS with nonsurgeon physicians at the scene on victims of refractory OHCA and that this technique can lead to neurologically intact survivors[38,40] (**Fig. 4**). In urban systems, a ground-based ECLS team delivery model may be effective, similar to that present in France. In suburban systems, it may be more effective to deliver the specialty ECLS team to the scene of the arrest by rotor-wing aircraft, similar to the current model of physician-staffed helicopter EMS teams in some countries in western Europe in response to major trauma incidents. Prehospital ECLS may not be feasible in less densely populated or rural areas, however, where the prevalence of refractory cardiac arrest patients that are candidates for ECLS precludes the sustainability of a specialty team. More research is needed to identify the appropriate patients for prehospital ECLS and to further

demonstrate clinical benefit. However, this concept is an intriguing emerging frontier in the science of OHCA resuscitation.

ULTRASOUND IMAGING IN OUT-OF-HOSPITAL CARDIAC ARREST MANAGEMENT

Point-of-care ultrasound examination has become commonplace in many emergency departments during the management of cardiac arrest.[41] Bedside ultrasound examination in the form of transthoracic echocardiography (TTE) may be able to assist in identifying reversible causes of pulseless electrical activity arrest, such as pericardial tamponade and massive pulmonary embolism, and may guide therapy such as pericardiocentesis or thrombolytic administration. TTE may also be of use as a prognostic tool to guide resuscitation efforts that often consume large amounts of time and resources.

Studies have yet to demonstrate a survival benefit to using TTE during cardiac arrest in the emergency department.[42–44] TTE does, however, provide information that can direct intervention outside of the standard Advanced Cardiac Life Support algorithm and has some prognostic utility in cases of visualized mechanical cardiac standstill, although these data are not conclusive.[43,44] The use of TTE for guidance during in-hospital cardiac arrest management is currently endorsed by the American College of Emergency Physicians.[45]

The use of TTE during the management of cardiac arrest is not without trade-offs. The act of acquiring transthoracic ultrasonographic views during pulse checks can be technically challenging and complicated by gastric insufflation from bag-valve-mask ventilation and from the positioning of defibrillator pads.[45–47] The use of TTE may result in prolonged pauses in chest compressions and a lower chest compression fraction.[44,48,49] Given that high-quality CPR is associated with improved survival,[10–13] prolonged pauses to obtain adequate ultrasonographic windows may be detrimental to victims of cardiac arrest.

Transesophageal echocardiography (TEE), facilitated by a small probe that is inserted into the esophagus after endotracheal intubation, has been shown to provide adequate images in most patients in a manner favorable to TTE.[47] TEE alleviates the ultrasonographic window challenges of TTE and can capture high-quality continuous images during both compressions and pulse checks without interfering with chest compressions or other procedures during cardiac arrest.[50–53] With decreasing equipment costs, TEE has become more accessible to emergency medicine providers.[54–56] The growth of TEE-guided cardiac

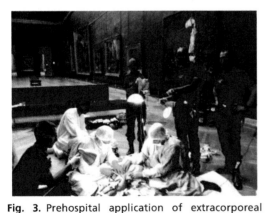

Fig. 3. Prehospital application of extracorporeal membrane oxygenation in the Louvre by the Service d'Aide Médicale Urgente (SAMU) in France. (*From* Lamhaut L, Hutin A, Deutsch J, et al. Extracorporeal Cardiopulmonary Resuscitation (ECPR) in the prehospital setting: an illustrative case of ECPR performed in the louvre museum. Prehosp Emerg Care 2017;21(3):387; with permission.)

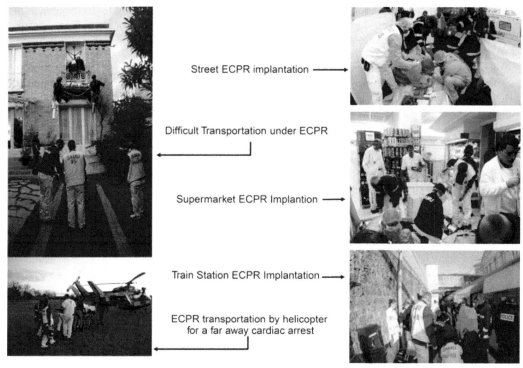

Street ECPR implantation ⟶

Difficult Transportation under ECPR ⌐

Supermarket ECPR Implantion ⟶

Train Station ECPR Implantation ⟶

ECPR transportation by helicopter
for a far away cardiac arrest

Fig. 4. Multiple instances of extracorporeal cardiopulmonary resuscitation (ECPR) by the Service d'Aide Médicale Urgente (SAMU) in France in different environments. (*From* Lamhaut L, Hutin A, Deutsch J, et al. Extracorporeal Cardiopulmonary Resuscitation (ECPR) in the prehospital setting: an illustrative case of ECPR performed in the louvre museum. Prehosp Emerg Care 2017;21(3):388; with permission.)

arrest resuscitation in some specialty centers has resulted in the American College of Emergency Physicians releasing guidelines regarding its use.[45,56]

TEE can facilitate modifying the location of chest compressions during closed chest CPR. Anatomic variation from patient to patient results in the area of maximal compression during CPR lying over the left ventricular outflow tract in as many as one-third of patients.[57,58] Positioning the hands over the ventricular side of the aortic valve during chest compressions during closed chest CPR seems to maximize stroke volume.[59] The focused use of TEE during cardiac arrest can be used to adjust hand positioning and, thus, the compression vector to augment resuscitative efforts in real time.[60,61] At the University of Utah, a small group of physicians perform TEE on cardiac arrest victims in the emergency department to adjust the positioning of a mechanical CPR device to optimize CPR mechanics.[26] Clinical outcomes data are still being collected.

As ultrasound-guided resuscitation experience and evidence grows, the next evolution in this technology may be the translation into the prehospital setting, because most cardiac arrests occur outside of the hospital. Several studies have demonstrated that paramedics can obtain adequate TTE images in the field during cardiac arrest resuscitation.[49,62–64] To our knowledge as of January 2018, no prehospital system has yet documented experience with guiding an OHCA with TEE. In the future, a specially trained advanced practice paramedic or possibly a prehospital physician could use TEE to guide OHCA resuscitation.[65]

UNMANNED AERIAL VEHICLES AND AUTOMATED EXTERNAL DEFIBRILLATOR DELIVERY

One emerging technology for the treatment of future victims of OHCA is beginning to take form. The concept of unmanned aerial vehicles, often referred to as drones, for the rapid delivery of AEDs to the scene of an OHCA for use by bystanders has begun testing.[66] Drone AED delivery is based on the concept that every minute in delay to defibrillation for a patient in cardiac arrest from a shockable rhythm decreases the probability of survival by roughly 10%.[67,68] Rapid arrival of an AED to the scene of an OHCA can dramatically improve survival.[69] Because decreasing time to defibrillation is one of the most important factors in survival from OHCA, many countries support extensive EMS systems with high capital and operational costs in part to reduce this time to first defibrillation.[70,71] Even within these systems, many first responders do not arrive on scene with defibrillation capability in those important first 5 to 10 minutes of arrest.[71]

The first solution to this problem has been the advent of public access AEDs (PADs), present in public places and businesses. PADs have been shown to improve survival for patients of OHCA[72–74]; however, they are not without their disadvantages. They may be difficult to find at the time of a cardiac arrest event, are occasionally located in businesses without 24/7 access, and are often not well-maintained or kept in organized up-to-date databases.[75] Moreover, most cardiac arrest events occur in the private setting, not in public, limiting the usefulness of PADs.[76] Owing to these factors, PADs historically have low use, with less than 3% of all OHCA events reporting that a PAD was applied.[75,76] Static deployment of public AEDs in the private setting and in more suburban and rural communities is also unlikely to be cost effective.[77–80]

Drone delivery of AEDs to the scene of an OHCA represents a novel way of reducing time to first defibrillation. This method may be able to overcome some of the barriers of AED availability and EMS response times in the private setting as well as in more suburban and rural areas.[81–83] Several feasibility studies on drone delivery of AEDs have been undertaken in Sweden, Canada, the United States, and Belgium[66,84–87] (**Fig. 5**). In Stockholm County, Sweden, geographic information system modeling demonstrated that in the rural setting, drone delivery of AEDs was likely to beat EMS arrival in 93% of cases and by a mean time of 19 minutes.[66,84] In Ontario, researchers have modeled a drone AED network that could deliver

an AED before EMS by up to 10 minutes in areas defined as rural in their study.[85] These times are likely to be clinically significant in the setting of a shockable OHCA event. These drone AED delivery networks may be cost effective,[87] and the drones might also be able to provide live video and audio transmission that could allow dispatchers to communicate with lay rescuers to improve and guide CPR.[82,83]

Drones capable of delivering AEDs to the scene of a patient in OHCA have been modeled and even patented by a number of groups[66,84,88] (**Fig. 6**). It is likely that autonomous, or mostly autonomous, drones will be the most effective.[89] However, there are many technical and regulatory barriers.[90] Future EMS systems using networks of drones capable of AED delivery may represent one of the next great advancement in the resuscitation of OHCA victims.

USE OF MOBILE TECHNOLOGY TO INCREASE BYSTANDER RESPONSE

Every Basic Life Support (BLS) class teaches students to call out for help. The human voice only travels so far. Telephones can reach assistance that is a distance away, but a specific number must be dialed. Technology enables targeted notification of those near an event that help is needed, thus digitizing the call for help. An early project in the Netherlands used a text message to alert trained rescuers, but the system did not have the geographic location of those responders. That system relied on sending alerts to many rescuers hoping that some would be close to the victim.[91] Later versions of the program, called Heartsafe Living – AED Alert, incorporated geographic location information of the phones.[71] Over more than

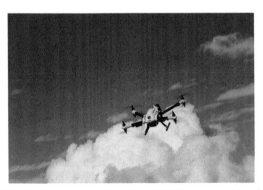

Fig. 5. An unmanned aerial vehicle/drone capable of carrying an automated external defibrillator used in Swedish feasibility studies. (*Courtesy of* Andreas Claesson, PhD, Floda, Sweden.)

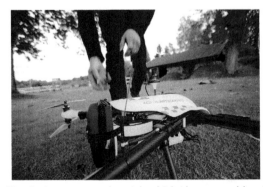

Fig. 6. An unmanned aerial vehicle/drone capable of carrying an automated external defibrillator used in Swedish feasibility studies. The automated external defibrillator is placed in the back of the drone for aerodynamic purposes. (*Courtesy of* PulsePoint Foundation. Pleasanton, CA; with permission.)

3 years, text message alerted responders delivered the first shock in 13% of shockable OHCA cases in parts of Holland.

In Stockholm, Sweden, the SMS-Lifesaver smartphone system notifies nearby lay rescuers of the need for CPR. A randomized trial showed that the SMS-Lifesaver system significantly increased the delivery of bystander CPR.[92] The developers of that system are planning a randomized trial to measure the impact of sending mobile lifesavers to fetch the nearest AED in addition to sending mobile lifesavers to start CPR without fetching an AED.[93] A similar, but nonrandomized study is ongoing in Seoul, South Korea.[94]

PulsePoint, an American smartphone technology to crowdsource bystander CPR and retrieve the nearest AED, was first implemented in California in January 2011. PulsePoint is available for download by anyone willing to do CPR and is active in communities that have integrated the technology within their 9-1-1 system. PulsePoint is also capable of notifying responders of nearby AEDs, if the AED is registered in the PulsePoint AED database (**Fig. 7**). By the end of 2017, PulsePoint had more than 60,000 registered AEDs ready for use by more than 1.25 million responders distributed throughout more than 2800 communities across the United States (**Fig. 8**).

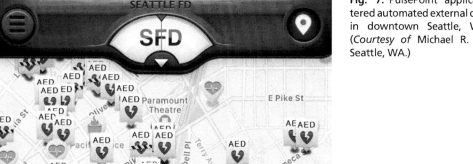

Fig. 7. PulsePoint application registered automated external defibrillators in downtown Seattle, Washington. (*Courtesy of* Michael R. Sayre, MD, Seattle, WA.)

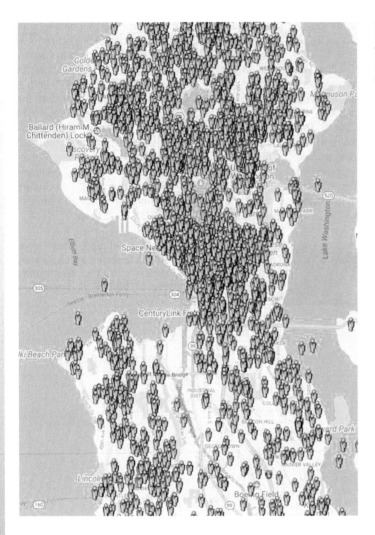

Fig. 8. Location of registered Pulse-Point application users in Seattle, Washington, in February 2018. (*Courtesy of* PulsePoint Foundation, Pleasanton, CA; with permission.)

PulsePoint, SMS-Lifesaver, and Heartsafe Living all require a witness to call emergency services (9-1-1 in North America) to activate the response. The GoodSAM system from the United Kingdom also offers a smartphone app that is integrated with emergency services dispatch to notify nearby responders of the need to CPR and an AED.[95] GoodSAM office staff verify the identities of those who sign up to respond. In addition, the GoodSAM system can be used to call emergency services using the smartphone app. In those cases, the exact location of the phone is available to emergency responders and other GoodSAM users nearby are activated directly.

In February 2017, PulsePoint launched a program in the United States to send verified responders to nearby cardiac arrests in residential settings.[96] Off-duty firefighters have been equipped with AEDs and are available to respond in suburban Portland, Oregon; areas around Spokane, Washington; and in Madison, Wisconsin. These technologies are still in early stages. When PulsePoint activates volunteer responders, only about 1 in 10 arrive at the scene of the emergency.[97] Many do not hear the notification or are unavailable to respond. Often volunteer responders are too far away from the event location to arrive before professional responders.[97]

The window of opportunity for smartphone enabled lifesavers may be quite short in a high-functioning EMS system. In some American cities, the median time interval from dispatcher recognition of a cardiac arrest to the arrival of the first professional responder at the patient is 6 minutes or less. Yet, in one-half of events, the time interval is more than 6 minutes. Those OHCA events with longer response intervals provide opportunities for smartphone equipped responders to have an impact by delivering CPR and an AED shock a minute or two earlier than the EMS system.

THE IMPACT OF WEARABLE TECHNOLOGY

About 70% of prehospital cardiac arrests with attempted resuscitation occur in the home.[98] Although loved ones are occasionally nearby, many of these arrests are classified as unwitnessed. Can technology fill the gap and recognize these arrests earlier than they otherwise would have been acknowledged? And once discovered, can there be treatment strategies put into place that can shorten important intervals in the resuscitation of these patients?

Although home telemetry monitoring has been available for some time, essentially as various forms and iterations of the Holter monitor, a true breakthrough in noninvasive cardiac monitoring has been elusive. Wrist-based devices have propagated through popular society and many of these track biometric properties including pulse rate and activity status in real time. Early versions of wrist-based devices have been found to be reliable to detect pulselessness in humans undergoing implantable defibrillator testing.[99] The early model studied by Rickard and colleagues[99] demonstrated a sensitivity of 99.9% and a specificity of 90.3% to detect pulselessness.

A major caveat exists with almost all smartwatch research to date; there has been little work done beyond feasibility studies. As King and Sarrafzadeh[100] note, 1119 smartwatch articles exist in the literature as of 2017, but only 27 are related to health care.[100] All of these studies have limited applications and are feasibility or usability studies. They were able to identify no randomized clinical trials performed on the efficacy of these devices.

One company has gone so far as to patent a process by which biometric, geospatial, and accelerometer data from a smartwatch and smartphone could be combined to contact a third party, possibly emergency services, and notify of a "care event," possibly an arrhythmia or cardiac arrest.[101] Once the cardiac arrest is detected and help is summoned, a second smartwatch on a lay rescuer could be used to optimize bystander CPR. This process has been studied and determined to be feasible.[102] The device in this report is able to detect and coach the wearer on various facets of CPR including depth and rate to align with international guideline recommendations.

As wearable devices become more and more common, sensor prices will decrease, and more people will have access to these potentially powerful tools. It is up to the generation of physicians who have grown from birth with these devices to harness their power to detect and alter the course of patients with OHCA.

SUMMARY

As discussed, there are a variety of future and emerging technologies that range from those focused on a narrow subset of refractory and/or recurrent OHCA patients, such as prehospital ECMO, to system wide technological advances including smartphone applications and wearable life detectors that could impact tens of thousands of people a year. One can imagine future systems of care using these technologies able to detect an OHCA event at the time of occurrence, notify nearby bystanders and EMS, and deliver an AED to the site by automated unmanned aerial vehicle. These advancements could be very impactful on survival from OHCA. There are approximately 365,000 OHCA events a year in the United States and roughly one-half receive a resuscitation attempt.[5,6] Twenty-five percent of these arrests are thought to originate in a shockable rhythm. Some portion of patients presenting initially in asystole are also likely to have initially been in a shockable rhythm that has deteriorated to asystole before EMS arrival. If we use these numbers, we can conservatively estimate approximately 45,000 patients that would benefit from immediate OHCA detection, earlier defibrillation, and improved bystander and EMS response. Currently, it is believed that fewer than 18,000 patients survive each year. These technologies have the ability to impact as many as 20,000 other patients annually in the United States alone.

Similar to the advances in cardiac arrest care that occurred in the 18th century and the improvements in survival that occurred in the second half of the 20th century, one or a combination of these emerging and future technologies will represent the next great leap in OHCA survival.

REFERENCES

1. Eisenberg M. History of the science of cardiopulmonary resuscitation. In: Ornato JP, Peberdy MA, editors. Cardiopulmonary resuscitation. Totowa (NJ): Humana Press Inc; 2005. p. 1–9.
2. Kouwenhoven WB, Jude JR, Knickerbocker GG. Closed-chest cardiac massage. JAMA 1960;173:1064–7.
3. Eisenberg M. Life in the balance: emergency medicine and the quest to reverse sudden death. New York: Oxford University Press; 1997.
4. Baskett TF, Baskett PJ. Frank Pantridge and mobile coronary care. Resuscitation 2001;48(2):99–104.
5. Benjamin E, Blaha M, Chiuve S, et al. Heart disease and stroke statistics—2017 update: a report from the American Heart Association. Circulation 2017;135(10):e146–603.

6. Girotra S, Diepen S, Nallamothu BK, et al. Regional variation in out-of-hospital cardiac arrest survival in the United States. Circulation 2016;133:2159–68.

7. Reynolds JC, Frisch A, Rittenberger JC, et al. Duration of resuscitation efforts and functional outcome after out-of-hospital cardiac arrest: when should we change to novel therapies? Circulation 2013; 128(23):2488–94.

8. Goto Y, Funada A, Goto Y. Relationship between the duration of cardiopulmonary resuscitation and favorable neurological outcomes after out-of-hospital cardiac arrest: a prospective, nationwide, population-based cohort study. J Am Heart Assoc 2016;5(3):e002819.

9. Olasveengen TM, Wik L, Steen PA. Quality of cardiopulmonary resuscitation before and during transport in out-of-hospital cardiac arrest. Resuscitation 2008;76(2):185–90.

10. Dumas F, Rea TD, Fahrenbruch C, et al. Chest compression alone cardiopulmonary resuscitation is associated with better long-term survival compared with standard cardiopulmonary resuscitation. Circulation 2013;127(4):435–41.

11. Wik L, Kramer-Johansen J, Myklebust H, et al. Quality of cardiopulmonary resuscitation during out-of-hospital cardiac arrest. JAMA 2005;293(3): 299–304.

12. Valenzuela TD, Kern KB, Clark LL, et al. Interruptions of chest compressions during emergency medical systems resuscitation. Circulation 2005; 112(9):1259–65.

13. Nolan JP, Hazinski MF, Aickin R, et al. Part 1: executive summary: 2015 international consensus on cardiopulmonary resuscitation and emergency cardiovascular care science with treatment Recommendations. Resuscitation 2015;95:e1–31.

14. Hallstrom A, Rea TD, Sayre MR, et al. Manual chest compression vs use of an automated chest compression device during resuscitation following out-of-hospital cardiac arrest: a randomized trial. JAMA 2006;295(22):2620–8.

15. Rubertsson S, Lindgren E, Smekal D, et al. Mechanical chest compressions and simultaneous defibrillation vs conventional cardiopulmonary resuscitation in out-of-hospital cardiac arrest: the LINC randomized trial. JAMA 2014;311(1): 53–61.

16. Wik L, Olsen J-A, Persse D, et al. Manual vs. integrated automatic load-distributing band CPR with equal survival after out of hospital cardiac arrest: the randomized CIRC trial. Resuscitation 2014; 85(6):741–8.

17. Perkins G, Lall R, Quinn T, et al. Mechanical versus manual chest compression for out-of-hospital cardiac arrest (PARAMEDIC): a pragmatic, cluster randomised controlled trial. Lancet 2015;385(9972):947–55.

18. Lyon RM, Crawford A, Crookston C, et al. The combined use of mechanical CPR and a carry sheet to maintain quality resuscitation in out-of-hospital cardiac arrest patients during extrication and transport. Resuscitation 2015;93:102–6.

19. Youngquist S, Hartsell S, McLaren D, et al. The use of prehospital variables to predict acute coronary artery disease in failed resuscitation attempts for out-of-hospital cardiac arrest. Resuscitation 2015; 92:82–7.

20. Dumas F, Bougouin W, Geri G, et al. Emergency percutaneous coronary intervention in post-cardiac arrest patients without ST-segment elevation pattern: insights from the PROCAT II registry. JACC Cardiovasc Interv 2016;9(10):1011–8.

21. Dumas F, Cariou A, Manzo-Silberman S, et al. Immediate percutaneous coronary intervention is associated with better survival after out-of-hospital cardiac arrest insights from the PROCAT (Parisian Region Out of Hospital Cardiac Arrest) registry. Circ Cardiovasc Interv 2010;3(3):200–7.

22. Libungan B, Dworeck C, Omerovic E. Successful percutaneous coronary intervention during cardiac arrest with use of an automated chest compression device: a case report. Ther Clin Risk Manag 2014; 10:255–7.

23. Ali A, Hothi SS, Cox D. Coronary intervention on a moving target: a case report and procedural considerations. J Invasive Cardiol 2013;25(8):E178–9.

24. Wagner H, Terkelsen CJ, Friberg H, et al. Cardiac arrest in the catheterisation laboratory: a 5-year experience of using mechanical chest compressions to facilitate PCI during prolonged resuscitation efforts. Resuscitation 2010;81(4):383–7.

25. Kennedy JH. The role of assisted circulation in cardiac resuscitation. JAMA 1966;197(8):615–8.

26. Youngquist ST, Scheppke KA, Pepe PE. Supportive technology in the resuscitation of out-of-hospital cardiac arrest patients. Curr Opin Crit Care 2017; 23(3):209–14.

27. Tonna JE, Selzman CH, Mallin MP, et al. Development and implementation of a comprehensive, multidisciplinary emergency department extracorporeal membrane oxygenation program. Ann Emerg Med 2017;70(1):32–40.

28. Bartos J, Voicu S, Matsuura T, et al. Role of epinephrine and extracorporeal membrane oxygenation in the management of ischemic refractory ventricular fibrillation. JACC Basic Transl Sci 2017;2(3):244–53.

29. Stub D, Bernard S, Pellegrino V, et al. Refractory cardiac arrest treated with mechanical CPR, hypothermia, ECMO and early reperfusion (the CHEER trial). Resuscitation 2015;86:88–94.

30. Yukawa T, Kashiura M, Sugiyama K, et al. Neurological outcomes and duration from cardiac arrest to the initiation of extracorporeal membrane

oxygenation in patients with out-of-hospital cardiac arrest: a retrospective study. Scand J Trauma Resusc Emerg Med 2017;25(1):95.

31. Kagawa E, Dote K, Kato M, et al. Should we emergently revascularize occluded coronaries for cardiac arrest? Rapid-response extracorporeal membrane oxygenation and intra-arrest percutaneous coronary intervention. Circulation 2012; 126(13):1605–13.

32. Sakamoto T, Morimura N, Nagao K, et al. Extracorporeal cardiopulmonary resuscitation versus conventional cardiopulmonary resuscitation in adults with out-of-hospital cardiac arrest: a prospective observational study. Resuscitation 2014;85(6): 762–8.

33. Yannopoulos D, Bartos J, Raveendran G, et al. Coronary artery disease in patients with out-of-hospital refractory ventricular fibrillation cardiac arrest. J Am Coll Cardiol 2017;70(9):1109–17.

34. Lamhaut L, Tea V, Raphalen JH, et al. Coronary lesions in refractory Out of Hospital Cardiac Arrest (OHCA) treated by Extra Corporeal Pulmonary Resuscitation (ECPR). Resuscitation 2017 [pii: S0300-9572(17)30797-9][Epub ahead of print].

35. Grunau B, Reynolds J, Scheuermeyer F, et al. Relationship between time-to-ROSC and survival in out-of-hospital cardiac arrest ECPR candidates: when is the best time to consider transport to hospital? Prehosp Emerg Care 2016;20(5):615–22.

36. Poppe M, Weiser C, Holzer M, et al. The incidence of "load and go" out-of-hospital cardiac arrest candidates for emergency department utilization of emergency extracorporeal life support: a one-year review. Resuscitation 2015;91:131–6.

37. Lamhaut L, Hutin A, Deutsch J, et al. Extracorporeal Cardiopulmonary Resuscitation (ECPR) in the prehospital setting: an illustrative case of ECPR performed in the louvre museum. Prehosp Emerg Care 2017;21(3):386–9.

38. Lamhaut L, Jouffroy R, Soldan M, et al. Safety and feasibility of prehospital extra corporeal life support implementation by non-surgeons for out-of-hospital refractory cardiac arrest. Resuscitation 2013; 84(11):1525–9.

39. Lamhaut L, Jouffroy R, Ellinger A, et al. A new therapeutic strategy for refractory cardiac arrest including prehospital ECMO: a comparison study. Am Heart Assoc 2015.

40. Lamhaut L, Hutin A, Puymirat E, et al. A pre-hospital Extracorporeal Cardio Pulmonary Resuscitation (ECPR) strategy for treatment of refractory out hospital cardiac arrest: an observational study and propensity analysis. Resuscitation 2017;117: 109–17.

41. Levitov A, Frankel H, Blaivas M, et al. Guidelines for the appropriate use of bedside general and cardiac ultrasonography in the evaluation of critically ill patients—part ii: cardiac ultrasonography. Crit Care Med 2016;44(6):1206.

42. Chardoli M, Heidari F, Rabiee H, et al. Echocardiography integrated ACLS protocol versus conventional cardiopulmonary resuscitation in patients with pulseless electrical activity cardiac arrest. Chin J Traumatol 2012;15(5):284–7.

43. Gaspari R, Weekes A, Adhikari S, et al. Emergency department point-of-care ultrasound in out-of-hospital and in-ED cardiac arrest. Resuscitation 2016;109:33–9.

44. Moskowitz A, Berg K. First do no harm: echocardiography during cardiac arrest may increase pulse check duration. Resuscitation 2017;119:A2–3.

45. Guidelines for the use of transesophageal echocardiography (TEE) in the ED for cardiac arrest. Ann Emerg Med 2017;70(3):442–5.

46. Parker MM, Cunnion RE, Parrillo JE. Echocardiography and nuclear cardiac imaging in the critical care unit. JAMA 1985;254:2935–9.

47. Heidenreich PA, Stainback RF, Redberg RF, et al. Transesophageal echocardiography predicts mortality in critically ill patients with unexplained hypotension. J Am Coll Cardiol 1995;26:152–8.

48. Veld M, Allison M, Bostick D, et al. Ultrasound use during cardiopulmonary resuscitation is associated with delays in chest compressions. Resuscitation 2017;119:95–8.

49. Reed M, Gibson L, Dewar A, et al. Introduction of paramedic led echo in life support into the prehospital environment: the PUCA study. Resuscitation 2017;112:65–9.

50. Miyake M, Izumi C, Takahashi S. Efficacy of transesophageal echocardiography in patients with cardiac arrest or shock. J Cardiol 2004;44(5):189–94.

51. Giraud R, Siegenthaler N, Schussler O, et al. The LUCAS 2 chest compression device is not always efficient: an echocardiographic confirmation. Ann Emerg Med 2015;65:23–6.

52. Wouw P, Koster R, Delemarre B, et al. Diagnostic accuracy of transesophageal echocardiography during cardiopulmonary resuscitation. J Am Coll Cardiol 1997;30(3):780–3.

53. Blaivas M. Transesophageal echocardiography during cardiopulmonary arrest in the emergency department. Resuscitation 2008;78:135–40.

54. Fair J, Tonna J, Ockerse P, et al. Emergency physician-performed transesophageal echocardiography for extracorporeal life support vascular cannula placement. Am J Emerg Med 2016;34(8): 1637–9.

55. Byars D, Tozer J, Joyce J, et al. Emergency physician-performed transesophageal echocardiography in simulated cardiac arrest. West J Emerg Med 2017;18(5):830–4.

56. Fair J, Mallin M, Mallemat H, et al. Transesophageal echocardiography: guidelines for point-of-care

applications in cardiac arrest resuscitation. Ann Emerg Med 2018;71(2):201–7.

57. Cha KC, Kim YJ, Shin HJ, et al. Optimal position for external chest compression during cardiopulmonary resuscitation: an analysis based on chest CT in patients resuscitated from cardiac arrest. Emerg Med J 2013;30:615–9.

58. Papadimitriou P, Chalkias A, Mastrokostopoulos A, et al. Anatomical structures underneath the sternum in healthy adults and implications for chest compressions. Am J Emerg Med 2013;31:549–55.

59. Hwang SO, Zhao PG, Choi HJ, et al. Compression of the left ventricular outflow tract during cardiopulmonary resuscitation. Acad Emerg Med 2009;16:928–33.

60. Arntfield R, Pace J, Hewak M, et al. Focused transesophageal echocardiography by emergency physicians is feasible and clinically influential: observational results from a novel ultrasound program. J Emerg Med 2016;50:286–94.

61. Anderson KL, Castaneda MG, Boudreau SM, et al. Left ventricular compressions improve hemodynamics in a swine model of out-of-hospital cardiac arrest. Prehosp Emerg Care 2017;21:272–80.

62. Prosen G, Križmarić M, Završnik J, et al. Impact of modified treatment in echocardiographically confirmed pseudo-pulseless electrical activity in out-of-hospital cardiac arrest patients with constant end-tidal carbon dioxide pressure during compression pauses. J Int Med Res 2010;38(4):1458–67.

63. Breitkreutz R, Price S, Steiger H, et al. Focused echocardiographic evaluation in life support and peri-resuscitation of emergency patients: a prospective trial. Resuscitation 2010;81(11):1527–33.

64. Aichinger G, Zechner P, Prause G, et al. Cardiac movement identified on prehospital echocardiography predicts outcome in cardiac arrest patients. Prehosp Emerg Care 2012;16(2):251–5.

65. Chenkin, Hockmann. LO23: a brief educational session is effective for teaching emergency medicine residents resuscitative transesophageal echocardiography. Can J Emerg Med 2017;19(S1):S35.

66. Claesson A, Bäckman A, Ringh M, et al. Time to delivery of an automated external defibrillator using a drone for simulated out-of-hospital cardiac arrests vs. emergency medical services. JAMA 2017;317(22):2332–4.

67. Valenzuela T, Roe D, Cretin S, et al. Estimating effectiveness of cardiac arrest interventions: a logistic regression survival model. Circulation 1997;96(10):3308–13.

68. Waalewijn R, Vos R, Tijssen J, et al. Survival models for out-of-hospital cardiopulmonary resuscitation from the perspectives of the bystander, the first responder, and the paramedic. Resuscitation 2001;51(2):113–22.

69. Nordberg P, Jonsson M, Forsberg S, et al. The survival benefit of dual dispatch of EMS and firefighters in out-of-hospital cardiac arrest may differ depending on population density – a prospective cohort study. Resuscitation 2015;90:143–9.

70. Ringh M, Jonsson M, Nordberg P, et al. Survival after public access defibrillation in Stockholm, Sweden – a striking success. Resuscitation 2015;91:1–7.

71. Zijlstra JA, Stieglis R, Riedijk F, et al. Local lay rescuers with AEDs, alerted by text messages, contribute to early defibrillation in a Dutch out-of-hospital cardiac arrest dispatch system. Resuscitation 2014;85:1444–9.

72. Aufderheide T, Hazinski M, Nichol G, et al. Community lay rescuer automated external defibrillation programs. Circulation 2006;113(9):1260–70.

73. Hazinski M, Idris A, Kerber R, et al. Lay rescuer automated external defibrillator ("public access defibrillation") programs. Circulation 2005;111(24):3336–40.

74. Hallstrom A, Oronato J, Weisfeldt M, et al. Public-access defibrillation and survival after out-of-hospital cardiac arrest. N Engl J Med 2004;351(7):637–46.

75. Sun C, Demirtas D, Brooks S, et al. Overcoming spatial and temporal barriers to public access defibrillators via optimization. J Am Coll Cardiol 2016;68(8):836–45.

76. Weisfeldt M, Sitlani C, Ornato J, et al. Survival after application of automatic external defibrillators before arrival of the emergency medical system evaluation in the resuscitation outcomes consortium population of 21 million. J Am Coll Cardiol 2010;55(16):1713–20.

77. Pell J, Walker A, Cobbe S. Cost-effectiveness of automated external defibrillators in public places: con. Curr Opin Cardiol 2007;22(1):5.

78. Winkle R. The effectiveness and cost effectiveness of public-access defibrillation. Clin Cardiol 2010;33(7):396–9.

79. Folke F, Gislason G, Lippert F, et al. Differences between out-of-hospital cardiac arrest in residential and public locations and implications for public-access defibrillation. Circulation 2010;122(6):623–30.

80. Siddiq A, Brooks S, Chan T. Modeling the impact of public access defibrillator range on public location cardiac arrest coverage. Resuscitation 2013;84(7):904–9.

81. Renkiewicz G, Hubble M, Wesley D, et al. Probability of a shockable presenting rhythm as a function of EMS response time. Prehosp Emerg Care 2014;18(2):224–30.

82. Floreano D, Wood R. Science, technology and the future of small autonomous drones. Nature 2015;521(7553):460–6.

83. Thiels C, Aho J, Zietlow S, et al. Use of unmanned aerial vehicles for medical product transport. Air Med J 2015;34(2):104–8.

84. Claesson A, Fredman D, Svensson L, et al. Unmanned aerial vehicles (drones) in out-of-hospital-cardiac-arrest. Scand J Trauma Resusc Emerg Med 2016;24(1):124.

85. Boutilier JJ, Brooks SC, Janmohamed A, et al. Optimizing a drone network to deliver automated external defibrillators. Circulation 2017;135(25):2454–65.

86. Pulver A, Wei R, Mann C. Locating AED enabled medical drones to enhance cardiac arrest response times. Prehosp Emerg Care 2016;20(3):378–89.

87. Van de Voorde P, Gautama S, Momont A, et al. The drone ambulance [A-UAS]: golden bullet or just a blank? Resuscitation 2017;116:46–8.

88. Patrick WG. Request apparatus for delivery of medical support implemented by UAV. U.S. Patent 9,307,383. 2016.

89. Dixon SR, Wickens CD, Chang D. Mission control of multiple unmanned aerial vehicles: a workload analysis. Hum Factors 2005;47(3):479–87.

90. Abrahamsen H. A remotely piloted aircraft system in major incident management: concept and pilot, feasibility study. BMC Emerg Med 2015;15(1):1–12.

91. Scholten A, van Manen J, van der Worp W, et al. Early cardiopulmonary resuscitation and use of automated external defibrillators by laypersons in out-of-hospital cardiac arrest using an SMS alert service. Resuscitation 2011;82:1273–8.

92. Ringh M, Rosenqvist M, Hollenberg J, et al. Mobile-phone dispatch of laypersons for CPR in out-of-hospital cardiac arrest. N Engl J Med 2015;372:2316–25.

93. Hollenberg J. Scandinavian AED and mobile bystander activation trial - NCT02992873.

94. Shin SD. Can Dispatcher-activated neighborhood access defibrillation and cardiopulmonary resuscitation improve survival of out-of hospital cardiac arrest? - NCT02010151. 2017.

95. Smith C, Wilson M, Ghorbangholi A, et al. The use of trained volunteers in the response to out-of-hospital cardiac arrest – the GoodSAM experience. Resuscitation 2017;121:123–6.

96. PulsePoint Foundation. Pilot program leverages off-duty professional firefighters, technology and defibrillators to save lives.

97. Brooks S, Simmons G, Worthington H, et al. The pulsepoint respond mobile device application to crowdsource basic life support for patients with out-of-hospital cardiac arrest: challenges for optimal implementation. Resuscitation 2016;98:20–6.

98. Fordyce CB, Hansen CM, Kraghoml K, et al. Association of public health initiatives with outcomes for out-of-hospital cardiac arrest at home and in public locations. JAMA Cardiol 2017;2(11):1226–35.

99. Rickard J, Ahmed S, Baruch M, et al. Utility of a novel watch-based pulse detection system to detect pulselessness in human subjects. Heart Rhythm 2011;8(12):1895–9.

100. King CE, Sarrafzadeh M. A survey of smartwatches in remote health monitoring. J Healthc Inform Res 2017. https://doi.org/10.1007/s41666-017-0012-7.

101. Hankey ME, Foster J, inventors. Apple Inc, applicant. Care event detection and alerts. Patent application number 14/849,427. Filed September 9, 2015.

102. Ahn C, Lee J, Oh J, et al. Effectiveness of feedback with a smartwatch for high-quality chest compressions during adult cardiac arrest: a randomized controlled simulation study. PLoS One 2017;12(4):e0169046.

Printed and bound by CPI Group (UK) Ltd, Croydon, CR0 4YY

03/10/2024

01040383-0019